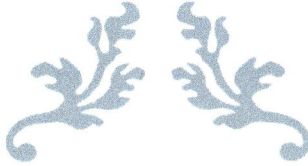

GO HOPEFUL

A Guide to Navigating Grief

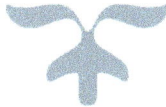

Finding Hope and Healing in the Shadow of Loss

BY JERRY WINRITE TOWNSEND

Library of Congress Control Number (LCCN): 9781966647775

ISBNs:
eBook: 978-1-966647-76-8
Paperback: 978-1-966647-77-5
Hardback: 978-1-966647-78-2

Published by:
Authors Publishing House
178 Broadway, 3rd Floor, #1343
New York, NY 10001, USA

Main Line: (855) 624-0155
Email: support@authorspublishinghouse.com

Table of Contents

Chapter 13: Creating a Long-Term Grief Management Plan.............. 99

Chapter 14: Ethical and Professional Considerations in Grief Support 108

Chapter 15: Integrating Go Hopeful into a Life of Fulfillment 116

Chapter 16: My Next Chapter After Grieving: A Reflective Guide.. 126

Worksheets 129

Foreword

One of the toughest processes of life is grief. It intrudes unwelcome, usually making us feel lost, broken and not knowing what the next thing is to do. The reason you may be holding this book is that you have probably suffered some kind of loss that has altered your world. First, I may say--you are not all alone.

In walking through my grief, I learned that grief is not a timeline, healing is not a straight line. There were days which were bearable, and there were days which were impossible. Gradually, however, I was taught that grief has little to do with getting over a loved one--it has much to do with learning how to continue to live with the memory of that person and how to find a means to resume life.

This book is to educate you on the various aspects of grief. Something we were never taught growing up. It provides soft advice, support and notices that you are not alone in your emotions. It is a reminder of the times when hope is so distant, and of the fact you can, even in the saddest moments of sorrow, find some light.

I hope that by reading these pages you will notice that you are no longer alone and that someone sees you, he understands you, and he is ready to support you. May this book help you to have the heart to meet the waves of grief, and the assurance that healing, in your own time and manner, is possible.

With compassion,

Jerry Winrite Townsend

Chapter 1
Understanding Grief and the Void

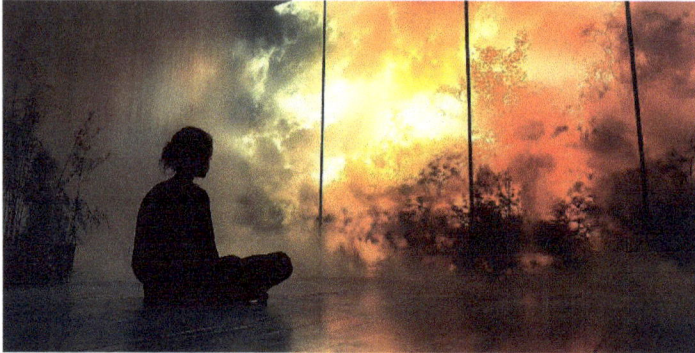

1.1   Defining Grief: Psychological and Emotional Dimensions

Grief is a natural response to losing someone or something deeply meaningful. It stirs a complex mix of emotions—sadness, anger, confusion, even moments of relief. Every person's grief follows its own rhythm, shaped by personality, history, and the depth of their connection to what was lost.

At times, grief feels like being caught in a storm: one moment calm, the next swept into unexpected waves of sorrow. Then, almost without warning, a small smile may appear at the memory of something once shared. These changes do not mean you are healing wrong—they are simply proof of love continuing to move through you.

Grief reaches beyond emotion; it touches both body and mind. Fatigue, difficulty focusing, and changes in appetite are common. These are not signs of weakness, but signs of caring deeply. Though it can feel isolating, grief often becomes a quiet invitation to connect—with yourself, with others who understand, and with the parts of your heart that are still learning how to live alongside loss.

The emptiness that follows loss can feel unbearable, but it reflects the depth of love that existed. This hollow space within you is not proof of something broken—it is evidence of something deeply cherished. Allowing yourself to feel its weight, without judgment or rush, is the first step toward healing.

1.2 The Concept of the Void in Loss and Mourning

When loss enters your life, it leaves behind a void—a silence that echoes through everything familiar. The world looks the same but feels completely changed. This space is more than absence; it is a shift in how life once felt whole. The routines, assumptions, and quiet certainties that once brought stability can suddenly seem fragile or distant.

The void unsettles, yet it also invites. Within its silence, questions about meaning and purpose arise: *Who am I now? How do I live without what I've lost?* These questions are not signs of despair but evidence of the mind and heart searching for balance after change.

Over time, the shape of the void shifts. Some days, it feels wide and consuming; other days, it softens into something you can carry. Accepting it as part of mourning does not mean surrendering to it. It means recognizing that emptiness has lessons of its own. Inside this space are traces of love, memory, and connection waiting to be honored rather than avoided.

Learning to sit quietly with the emptiness can become an act of healing. When we stop fighting the silence, we begin to understand what it holds—reminders of love, resilience, and the courage it takes to feel deeply.

The void also becomes a mirror for transformation. It can change how we see ourselves, prompting deeper empathy and appreciation for life. Many discover that grief does not simply wound—it refines. The pain becomes softer over time, not because we forget, but because we learn how to live with it.

Simple rituals can help transform the void from something feared into something sacred: lighting a candle, writing a letter, or revisiting a place that carries meaning. These small gestures remind us that love still exists, even in absence.

1.3   Common Myths and Misconceptions About Grief

Grief often carries invisible expectations—quiet beliefs about what healing "should" look like. These myths, passed down through culture or conversation, can make the grieving process harder by creating pressure or guilt. Understanding and releasing them allows us to move through grief with more patience and compassion.

Myth 1: Grief has a timeline.

One of the most persistent myths is that grief should be over within a specific time frame—a year, six months, or even less. You may hear others say, *"You should be feeling better by now."* But grief doesn't measure itself in weeks or months. It comes and goes like the tide, calm one day and heavy the next. Healing is not about speed; it's about honesty—allowing each emotion the time it needs.

Myth 2: If I'm not crying, I'm not grieving.

Tears are one expression of grief, but they are not the only one. Some people grieve quietly through thought, art, prayer, or stillness. Others show it through action or caretaking. The absence of visible emotion doesn't mean a lack of love—it simply means the heart has chosen another language.

Myth 3: Moving on means forgetting.

Healing is not about letting go of love but about letting go of pain's control. To "move forward" is not to erase the past; it's to carry it differently. The person or experience you lost remains part of your story—woven into how you see the world and how you care for others. Healing honors that connection by allowing it to live on in new ways.

Myth 4: Strong people don't grieve deeply.

True strength is not the absence of emotion; it's the willingness to feel. It takes courage to admit pain, to cry, and to reach out for help.

Holding back may seem brave, but it only builds walls that isolate. Strength is found in honesty, not endurance alone.

Myth 5: Grief follows a neat set of stages.

While models like the "five stages of grief" can be helpful for understanding emotion, real grief is rarely so orderly. Feelings may overlap or return when least expected. You might feel acceptance one day and disbelief the next. This ebb and flow isn't failure—it's a natural rhythm of healing, where progress and pain often travel together.

Myth 6: Staying busy helps you heal faster.

Distraction may ease the pain for a while, but constant motion leaves grief unaddressed. Healing comes from moments of stillness—those quiet times when we allow tears, memories, and reflection to surface. Resting, remembering, and simply breathing through difficult moments are not signs of weakness; they are signs of courage.

Myth 7: My grief isn't as valid as someone else's.

There's no scale for sorrow. Whether you've lost a loved one, a dream, a relationship, or a stage of life, your pain deserves acknowledgment. Comparing your grief to another's only deepens the loneliness. Each loss changes the world in a personal way, and every loss is worthy of compassion.

Myth 8: Time heals all wounds.

Time alone doesn't heal—it simply moves forward. What heals is how we live within that time: through reflection, connection, and kindness toward ourselves. With gentle care, time becomes a companion that helps soften grief's sharp edges and makes space for a quieter kind of love to grow.

A More Honest View of Healing

Grief doesn't follow rules, nor does it end at a finish line. It becomes a companion that changes shape over time—a reminder not only of what was lost but also of how deeply we can love. Letting go of these myths opens the way to a more authentic experience of healing—one that allows sorrow and hope to coexist, each giving meaning to the other.

❀ Summary of Core Takeaways

1. Grief is natural, multifaceted, and deeply personal.
2. Emotional fluctuations are part of healing, not signs of weakness.
3. The void after loss reflects both pain and love.
4. Facing the emptiness creates growth and resilience.
5. Healing unfolds in its own time through patience, rituals, and compassion.

Chapter 2
The Psychology of Embracing Loss

2.1 The Stages of Grief: An Evidence-Based Approach

Grief is not a single feeling or a single road. It's an ever-changing landscape where love and pain meet in unfamiliar ways. One day you might feel steady, even peaceful, and the next you find yourself undone by a memory, a smell, or a song that opens the wound again. This rhythm of calm and chaos is part of grief's strange language.

When someone or something precious is gone, the world doesn't look the same. The simplest routines—pouring coffee, setting the table, hearing laughter in another room—can feel hollow. Even breathing can feel like an effort when life has lost its familiar shape. Grief rearranges everything; it touches sleep, appetite, memory, and even your sense of who you are.

And yet, this landscape isn't barren. Within the pain lies the evidence of love—the deeper the bond, the stronger the ache. Grief is proof that what was lost truly mattered. Understanding this can shift the question from *"Why am I hurting so much?"* to *"Why did I love so deeply?"* That change in perspective, though small, begins to soften the edges of despair.

2.2 Cognitive and Emotional Responses to Loss

Grief rarely moves in straight lines; it ebbs and flows like the tide. Emotions arrive uninvited—sometimes crashing, sometimes whispering.

Denial often appears first, not as ignorance but as protection. It's the mind's gentle shield, giving you space to breathe when the truth feels too large to bear. You may find yourself expecting a phone call that will never come, or turning to speak to someone who isn't there. This isn't denial of reality—it's the heart trying to delay heartbreak until it feels safe enough to face it.

Then comes **anger**, sharp and consuming. You might feel angry at circumstances, at fate, at yourself, or even at the one who is gone. Anger is love wearing armor—it says, *"This mattered. I am not ready to let it go."* When treated with understanding rather than guilt, anger can become a force of clarity and renewal.

Bargaining often follows, filled with "if only" and "what if." It's the mind's attempt to regain control after the world has stopped making sense. Bargaining can sound like prayer or regret or endless replaying of the past. It reveals the longing to rewrite what cannot be rewritten—a sign not of weakness, but of love searching for safety.

Then comes the deep, quiet weight of **sadness**. It may feel endless, heavy as fog. This is the moment when the loss truly settles in—the reality that what once was will never be again. But even in this darkness, there are small lights: the warmth of memory, the kindness of a friend, the tender realization that feeling deeply means you are still alive to love.

Eventually, **acceptance** begins to weave itself gently through the sorrow. It is not a single moment of closure but a slow awakening. Acceptance means you start to live alongside the absence instead of fighting it. You begin to carry your love differently—not as pain, but as quiet remembrance.

These emotions are not steps to be checked off. They come and go, overlap, and return when you least expect them. Some days you might feel strong; other days you may feel as though you've gone backward. But grief doesn't move backward—it circles closer to peace each time it returns.

How Loss Affects the Mind and Heart

Grief doesn't live only in emotion; it also takes up residence in the body and mind. The brain, trying to make sense of the unthinkable, can spin in loops—replaying the last conversation, re-examining choices, searching for reason in something that feels unreasonable. You might forget where you set your keys, lose track of days, or stare blankly at simple tasks. This fog isn't failure; it's your mind protecting you from overload.

Physically, grief can show up as exhaustion, tightness in the chest, stomach upset, or feeling unusually restless. The body grieves too—it carries the weight of absence.

Emotionally, the heart moves through countless colors: sorrow, guilt, relief, fear, and even moments of laughter that surprise you. Some days you might feel grateful for what you had; others, angry that it ended. These contradictions can feel confusing, but they are signs of healing—the heart stretching to hold all sides of truth.

You may also notice subtle spiritual or existential shifts. Loss makes us question meaning, purpose, and fairness. For some, it shakes faith; for others, it deepens it. In both cases, it invites a deeper reflection on what it means to be alive, to love, and to keep going.

When the mind feels overwhelmed, gentleness is medicine. Write a few words in a journal. Sit in silence. Let the tears come, then rest. Healing happens in small, almost invisible moments when you stop demanding answers and simply allow yourself to be.

2.3　The Role of Resilience and Post-Traumatic Growth

Resilience doesn't mean being unshaken; it means learning to stand again after the wave passes. It's the slow rebuilding of trust in life's goodness, even when you've seen its cruelty.

You build resilience through the smallest acts of care: getting dressed when you'd rather stay in bed, letting sunlight touch your face, accepting a friend's invitation, taking a walk, saying "yes" to one small thing today. These gestures seem simple, but they whisper life back into the spaces grief emptied.

Resilience also means letting yourself break when you need to. There will be days when tears come easily, when strength feels far away. Those moments don't erase progress—they are part of it. Every tear is evidence that your heart is still beating, still capable of love.

Over time, resilience becomes a quiet faith in yourself. It says, *I can feel this pain and still find beauty. I can remember what I lost and still move toward what remains.*

Growth Beyond the Pain

Grief may begin as darkness, but it can also become a deep teacher. In its shadow, we often discover unexpected gifts: compassion, humility, patience, and a clearer sense of what matters most.

Some people find that their capacity for empathy expands. They listen more gently, love more freely, and judge less quickly. Others find new purpose—a cause, a craft, or a way of helping others who are hurting. These transformations don't erase pain, but they give it meaning. They turn suffering into soil from which something living can grow.

Over time, the relationship with loss changes. The sharp ache becomes a tender scar—something that still twinges but no longer defines you. The memories remain, but they start to bring warmth instead of only tears. You begin to carry love not as a wound but as a legacy.

Healing does not mean forgetting. It means remembering with peace, allowing the heart to hold both joy and sorrow at once. That balance—the coexistence of what was and what still is—is where healing truly lives.

🌸 Summary of Core Takeaways

1. The five stages of grief describe possibilities, not rules.
2. Denial, anger, and bargaining serve as natural defenses that allow adaptation.
3. Depression and acceptance mark deeper processing and integration.
4. Cognitive and emotional chaos are normal as the mind reorganizes around loss.
5. Resilience grows through small actions, community, and self-compassion.
6. Post-traumatic growth transforms suffering into insight and renewed purpose.
7. Healing means carrying the loss with love—not leaving it behind.

Chapter 3
Cultural and Spiritual Perspectives on Grief

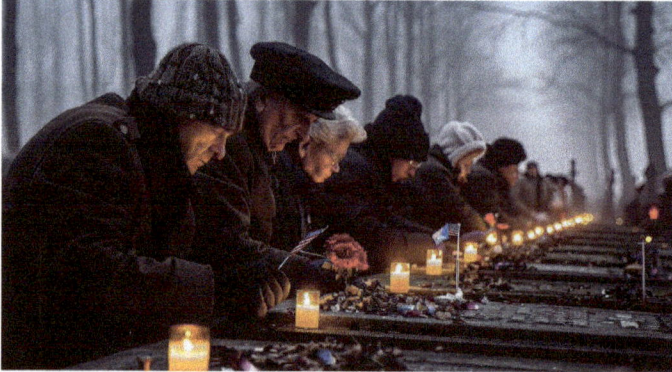

3.1   Cultural Rituals and Practices for Mourning

Cultural rituals offer individuals a way to cope with the sorrow of losing a loved one, serving as a structured approach to express grief and honor the deceased. Different cultures have developed unique practices that provide comfort during these difficult times. For example, in Mexico, Día de los Muertos, or the Day of the Dead, is a vibrant celebration where families create altars and offer food, flowers, and mementos to deceased relatives.

This festival allows people to remember their loved ones joyfully, blending remembrance with celebration. In Jewish culture, the practice of sitting shiva involves mourning for seven days, where the bereaved are supported by friends and family, creating a communal environment for sharing grief and memories.

3.2   Spiritual Beliefs and Their Influence on Healing

Spiritual beliefs often serve as a foundation for comfort and meaning during the grieving process. When faced with loss, many find solace in understanding that death may not be an end but a transition to another form of existence. Ideas about the soul, an afterlife, or a greater universal plan help create a sense of peace amid emotional turmoil.

For some, prayer, meditation, or rituals associated with their faith offer ways to connect with the departed and express their grief in a structured manner. These practices can quiet the mind, ease feelings of loneliness, and reinforce hope that loved ones remain present in some way beyond physical separation. Different traditions provide unique frameworks to interpret loss, shaping how individuals move through healing.

In some cultures, mourning rituals encourage gathering, sharing memories, and openly expressing sorrow, which helps people feel supported rather than isolated. Other spiritual systems emphasize acceptance and release, guiding mourners to find inner calm by trusting the natural flow of life and death. These perspectives influence not only emotional responses but also physical healing, as faith can reduce stress hormones and enhance mental resilience.

By trusting in something beyond the immediate pain, bereaved individuals often regain a sense of purpose and direction. Spirituality also influences how healing is practiced personally and within communities. Some rely on blessings, anointing, or energy healing, believing these acts restore balance between body, mind, and spirit.

Traditional ceremonies, such as smudging or chanting, are thought to cleanse pain and invite positive energy. This approach to healing respects the whole person, recognizing grief as more than an emotional experience, it is a shift that touches every part of being. The integration of spiritual care alongside medical or psychological support often creates a more nurturing environment, acknowledging the grieving person's need for both practical help and deeper meaning.

Many find that embracing their spiritual beliefs during times of grief encourages reflection on life's fragility and value. Recognizing loss as part of a larger cycle can foster gratitude for shared moments and inspire a commitment to live with greater intention. The process of healing becomes not just about overcoming sadness but also about growth and transformation.

Keeping rituals or spiritual practices alive, even in subtle ways, can maintain a connection to the person who has passed and provide ongoing comfort. Engaging with these beliefs allows grief to be experienced fully without losing hope or identity. A helpful insight for those navigating grief through spirituality is to honor what feels authentic and meaningful.

It's okay to adapt traditional practices or find new ways to express faith that resonate personally. Healing is rarely a straight path, and spiritual beliefs can offer both answers and questions that encourage exploration. Whether through quiet moments of prayer, sharing stories, or participating in community ceremonies, these actions invite healing energy and create a safe space for grief to unfold naturally.

3.3 Integrating Cultural and Spiritual Resources in Grief Support

Cultural and spiritual beliefs play a central role in how people understand and process grief. These beliefs influence what they see as appropriate ways to mourn, honor, and remember loved ones. For example, some cultures emphasize celebrating life through rituals and gatherings, while others focus on quiet reflection and prayer.

Spiritual beliefs often provide frameworks for making sense of loss, offering explanations like the soul's journey or life after death. Recognizing these core beliefs helps caregivers approach grief support with sensitivity, respecting what matters deeply to each person. Understanding these perspectives can also prevent misunderstandings and foster trust, creating a more meaningful connection during difficult times.

Integrating cultural and spiritual resources into grief support involves acknowledging the diverse traditions and practices that individuals cherish. This means asking open-ended questions about their backgrounds and beliefs and listening carefully to their stories. For some, participating in specific rituals— such as lighting candles, reciting prayers, or performing customary ceremonies— can bring comfort and a sense of connection.

Others might find solace in cultural symbols, music, or storytelling that honor their heritage. Recognizing and respecting these elements can help create a supportive environment in which the grieving person feels seen and understood. It also allows support providers to tailor assistance to fit the person's unique spiritual and cultural framework, making healing a more personal and respectful experience.

Incorporating cultural and spiritual considerations into grief support can also mean encouraging practices that resonate personally, whether that involves prayer, meditation, or traditional rituals. It's helpful to explore what these practices mean to the individual, rather than assuming a one-size-fits-all approach. For example, offering space for prayer or meditation, or suggesting ways to incorporate cultural objects into remembrance activities, can be meaningful.

Sometimes, simply acknowledging and validating the significance of these practices helps bereaved persons feel empowered in their coping process. Supporting their choice to engage with certain rituals or spiritual expressions reinforces respect and acceptance, which can be particularly healing amidst their ongoing journey through grief.

Understanding our different beliefs around grief.

Different faiths approach grief in unique ways, shaped by their beliefs about life, death, the soul, and the afterlife. These traditions offer rituals, theology, and community support that help people process loss. Below is a look at how **major world religions** treat grief with sensitivity to both their doctrines and how individuals may experience them in real life.

Christianity

Beliefs: Life after death, resurrection, heaven, eternal union with God.

Grief Response:

- Grief is seen as natural, but not hopeless: "We do not grieve as those who have no hope"

  (1 Thessalonians 4:13).

- Prayer, scripture, and rituals (like funerals and memorial services) offer comfort.
- Emphasis on the **hope of reunion** in heaven.
- In some traditions (especially Catholicism), prayers for the dead are common (e.g., the Rosary, Requiem Mass).

Emotional Tone: Hopeful sorrow. God is seen as a comforter, and the grieving person may find peace in surrender or in trusting God's larger plan.

Judaism

Beliefs: Life is sacred; death is part of God's plan. Beliefs about the afterlife vary, but often focus more on living well in the present.

Grief Response:

- Structured mourning periods: **Shiva (7 days), Shloshim (30 days), and Yahrzeit (yearly remembrance).**
- Community plays a huge role—visits, meals, and prayers (e.g., *Kaddish*).
- Mourning is seen as a commanded, communal, and sacred act.
- Expression of grief is allowed and even encouraged—anger, sadness, questioning.

Emotional Tone: Grounded, communal, and honest. Ritual helps process pain without rushing it.

Islam

Beliefs: Life and death are part of God's will. There is an afterlife, and the soul continues.

Grief Response:

- Immediate burial is important; mourners often say *"Inna lillahi wa inna ilayhi raji'un"* ("We belong to God and to Him we return").
- Mourning periods vary (3 days for most, 4 months, and 10 days for windows).

- Excessive wailing or despair is discouraged. Patience and trust in God's wisdom are emphasized.
- Prayers and recitation of the Qur'an for the deceased are common.

Emotional Tone: Surrender, patience, faith. Grief is acknowledged but balanced by deep submission to God's will.

Hinduism

Beliefs: Reincarnation, karma, the soul (Atman) is eternal. Death is part of the soul's journey.

Grief Response:

- Rituals focus on helping the soul transition—e.g., cremation, 10–13 days of mourning, **Shraddha** (memorial rituals).
- Grief is acknowledged but not clung to. Too much attachment is seen as binding the soul.
- Chanting, offerings, and recitation of sacred texts are common.

Emotional Tone: Acceptance, detachment, and spiritual support for the soul's journey.

Buddhism

Beliefs: Impermanence (arnica), karma, rebirth. Attachment causes suffering.

Grief Response:

- Death is a natural part of the cycle of existence (samsara).
- Mourning practices include meditation, chanting (e.g., for a peaceful rebirth), and mindful grieving.
- Grief is not denied but **transformed** through awareness, compassion, and letting go.
- In some traditions, there is a 49-day period (bardo) between death and rebirth, during which rituals help guide the deceased.

Emotional Tone: Mindful, compassionate, introspective. The emphasis is on non-attachment and inner peace.

Indigenous and Traditional Spiritualities

These vary widely across cultures but often include:

- **Connection to ancestors**
- **Cyclic view of life and death**
- **Rituals and storytelling** as part of healing
- Grief is often processed communally, through ceremony, dance, art, or time in nature.

Emotional Tone: Integrative grief connects the mourner to the spiritual realm, nature, and community.

Secular or Spiritual-But-Not-Religious Approaches

Many people who don't follow a specific religion still draw on spiritual ideas:

- Belief in the **energy or memory** of the deceased living on.

- Use of **rituals** (like lighting candles, journaling, nature walks).

- Grief as a **transformative** spiritual experience, even without specific beliefs in God or an afterlife.

Summary Table:

Faith	Afterlife Belief	Grief Tone	Key Rituals/Practices
Christianity	Heaven, resurrection	Hopeful sorrow	Funerals, prayer, scripture, communion
Judaism	Varies; focus on life now	Honest, communal	Shiva, Kaddish, yearly remembrance
Islam	Heaven, soul continues	Surrender, patience	Immediate burial, Qur'an recitation
Hinduism	Rebirth, karma	Acceptance, detachment	Cremation, Shraddha, chanting
Buddhism	Rebirth, impermanence	Mindful, peaceful	Meditation, chanting, bardo rituals
Indigenous	Ancestor connection, cycles	Communal, sacred	Ceremonies, storytelling, offerings

🌸 Summary of Core Takeaways

1. Cultural rituals bring structure, meaning, and shared support to grief.

2. Spiritual beliefs transform death into continuity, anchoring hope.

3. Community presence turns isolation into connection and comfort.

4. Faith practices—prayer, reflection, ritual—calm the mind and body.

5. Authentic and adaptable expressions of belief strengthen resilience.

6. Sensitivity to cultural and spiritual values enhances meaningful care.

7. Healing is holistic: emotional, physical, cultural, and spiritual renewal working together.

Chapter 4
Developing a Personal Grief Narrative

4.1   Guided Techniques for Storytelling and Reflection

Storytelling serves as a powerful tool for individuals navigating their grief. Through the act of storytelling, people can shape and understand their personal narratives surrounding loss. The journey of grieving can be overwhelming, filled with a range of emotions that often feel chaotic or confusing.

By engaging in storytelling, it becomes possible to create a more coherent narrative that helps process these feelings. Mindfulness plays a significant role in this process, encouraging individuals to reflect honestly on their experiences and emotions. This honesty can foster deeper understanding and gradually lead to healing, as one begins to make sense of their grief in a personal context.

Practical techniques can aid in this reflective storytelling process. Journaling is a particularly effective method. One might begin by exploring specific prompts, such as "What do I most miss about my loved one" or "Can I describe a moment when I felt their presence." These questions not only encourage thought but also allow for a deeper exploration of emotions tied to memories. Visualization exercises can complement journaling.

For instance, an individual may close their eyes and envision a peaceful place they shared with the lost loved one. This type of mental imagery can evoke strong feelings and help articulate thoughts that might not come easily. Reflective questions, such as "What lessons have I learned from this loss." or "How has this experience changed me." can guide individuals toward a clearer understanding of their grief and encourage a deeper connection to their narrative. The integration of these techniques into daily life can nurture a more profound engagement with those feelings.

Whether through writing or visual reflection, the goal is to create a space where emotions can be expressed freely and safely. Through storytelling, grief can transform from a confusing whirlwind into a narrative that is not only understood but also celebrated as part of a life lived fully. Embracing one's grief story offers a unique opportunity to honor memories while fostering resilience.

Take a few moments each day to write down thoughts or feelings. Allow the words to flow without judgment, knowing that this practice can provide clarity and comfort in difficult times.

4.2   Transforming Pain into Personal Meaning

Grief often feels like an unbearable weight that leaves us struggling to find purpose in the midst of suffering. The process of reframing grief means shifting how we view loss, not by ignoring the pain but by allowing it to reveal deeper parts of ourselves. This does not happen quickly or easily; grief is complex and unique for everyone.

When we start to look beyond the immediate pain, we can begin to recognize how grief shapes our understanding of life, connection, and what matters most to us. It is through this slow and thoughtful reconsideration of loss that personal meaning begins to emerge, sometimes in surprising ways. Instead of focusing only on what has been taken away, reframing grief invites us to notice what remains or what can still grow.

For example, some people find that their grief deepens empathy towards others, inspiring acts of kindness they might not have felt before. Others discover a new sense of strength or clarity about their priorities. These changes don't erase heartache but create space for a renewed sense of purpose.

By accepting grief as part of our story, not just a moment of pain but a chapter that informs who we are, meaning surfaces naturally over time. This shift helps form a bridge from despair toward a more hopeful outlook. One way to begin transforming emotional pain is to give yourself permission to fully experience your feelings without judgment or pressure to move on quickly.

Emotions like sadness, anger, and confusion are natural responses to loss, and sitting with these feelings can reveal layers of self-awareness. Writing about your experience, whether in a journal or in letters to the person you lost, can be a powerful tool for processing complex emotions and organizing your thoughts. This practice often leads to insights about your resilience and values that might have been overlooked amid the initial shock.

Another helpful approach is to engage in small, consistent acts of self-care that honor your needs. This might include gentle movement, spending time in nature, or creating quiet moments for reflection. These activities provide grounding and help restore a sense of balance, which is essential when grief destabilizes everyday life.

Connecting with supportive people who listen without trying to fix your feelings can also nurture healing. Sometimes growth emerges from sharing your story and recognizing you are not alone in your pain. As you continue this process, you may notice gradual shifts—not just in your mood but in how you see yourself and your capacity to face challenges.

Finding meaning in pain often requires patience and openness to change. Setting small, achievable goals related to personal growth can guide your journey. Whether it involves learning something new, helping others, or exploring creative outlets, these efforts encourage self-discovery and remind you of your inner strength.

Remember that transforming grief is not about leaving the past behind but weaving it into your present in a way that brings value and understanding. Allowing time, kindness, and intentional action to guide you can turn even the deepest pain into a source of wisdom and renewed purpose.

4.3 Identifying and Challenging Unhelpful Narratives

Many people carrying grief tend to hold onto certain stories or beliefs that can slow down their healing process. These stories often paint a picture of loss as an unchangeable, overwhelming force. For example, believing that life will never be the same or that the pain will last forever can create a feeling of hopelessness.

Such narratives set up the idea that feeling better is impossible, which can cause people to withdraw or avoid facing their emotions. Recognizing these ideas as common but unhelpful is a first step toward changing how you approach grief. When these beliefs take hold, they can prevent healing by making the pain seem endless or insurmountable, trapping individuals in a cycle of sadness and frustration.

Unhelpful grief stories often include notions like I should have done more or It's my fault. These beliefs can lead to feelings of guilt and self-blame that distort reality and create unnecessary suffering. Others might think I'll never be able to smile again, which discourages trying to find moments of happiness.

These narratives also tend to generalize the pain, making it seem all-consuming and defining one's entire life. Such thoughts can cause a person to cling to despair, avoiding ways to adapt or find new meaning. Recognizing these patterns helps in understanding that these stories are not facts but mental constructs that can be challenged and changed.

The impact of these narratives extends beyond emotional pain. They can influence daily decisions, relationships, and even physical health by fueling ongoing stress and sadness. When the story becomes, "I am forever broken," it can inhibit a person from even attempting to rebuild parts of their life.

These stories become self-fulfilling prophecies if left unchecked, solidifying a sense of helplessness. Understanding that these are stories rather than truths opens the door to questioning their validity. This awareness is essential because it allows space for alternative, more compassionate narratives to take hold, helping individuals move gradually toward healing.

The first step in challenging unhelpful grief stories is becoming aware of them. Pay attention to the thoughts that tend to arise during moments of sadness or stress. Notice when your mind is repeating ideas like this, pain will never go away, or I can't live without them.

Writing down these thoughts can make it easier to see and evaluate. Once identified, question the truth of these stories. Ask yourself, "Is this really true." or "What evidence do I have that contradicts this belief." Often, you will find that these ideas are exaggerated or based on assumptions rather than facts. After examining these beliefs, try replacing them with more balanced and realistic thoughts.

Swap "I'll never feel better" for "Sadness helps me heal, and pain fades with time." This process doesn't mean forcing yourself to be joyful but rather acknowledging feelings while maintaining hope. Practicing self-compassion is also crucial; recognizing that grief is a natural response and not a sign of weakness.

Engaging in activities that promote mindfulness, such as breathing exercises or gentle movement, can help you step back from these stories. Over time, consistently questioning and reframing unhelpful beliefs weakens their hold, creating space for new, healthier narratives to develop. Trying simple exercises like challenging negative thoughts whenever they come up can make a difference.

For example, if you catch yourself thinking, "I'll never be happy again," pause and consider alternative perspectives. Remind yourself of moments when you felt joy or hope, even if small. It can be helpful to talk about these thoughts with a trusted friend, therapist, or support group.

Sometimes just voicing unhelpful beliefs makes it easier to see their flaws. Remember that changing stories takes time and patience. Small shifts in how you interpret your experiences can gradually lead to a more compassionate view of yourself and your journey through grief.

Incorporating these practices into daily life helps build resilience against harmful narratives. Keep a journal of thoughts and how you challenge them. Over time, you'll notice patterns and become more skilled at noticing when old stories start to reappear.

This awareness is a powerful tool to support ongoing healing because it puts you in control of your inner narrative. Rather than letting grief stories dictate your feelings, you start to create a space where more gentle, realistic, and hopeful stories can grow. This shift doesn't erase pain but changes how you relate to it, helping you move forward at your own pace.

🌸 Summary of Core Takeaways

1. Storytelling and reflection transform chaos into clarity.
2. Mindfulness and journaling cultivate self-awareness and healing.
3. Meaning making turns grief into growth and compassion.
4. Self-care and connection rebuild strength and hope.
5. Challenging unhelpful beliefs frees the heart from despair.
6. Reframing the grief story empowers renewal and peace.

Chapter 5
Practical Strategies for Facing the Void

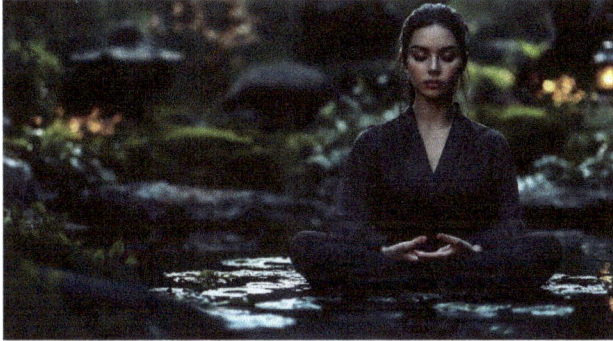

5.1   Mindfulness and Acceptance-Based Approaches

Mindfulness is a powerful tool for those navigating the turbulent waters of grief. It encourages you to focus on the here and now, helping to counteract the overwhelming feelings that can arise when remembering a loved one. One effective technique is mindful breathing. This involves paying attention to your breath, noticing the sensations as you inhale and exhale.

You can practice this anywhere, whether sitting quietly in your room or taking a walk outside. Concentrating on your breath can ground you, providing a brief respite from the emotional storm. Another approach is body scanning, which involves mentally checking in with different parts of your body. By focusing your attention on areas of tension or discomfort, you can release some of the physical manifestations of grief, promoting relaxation.

Observing your thoughts without judgment is another mindfulness practice. When you experience feelings related to grief, such as sadness or anger, try to acknowledge them without getting swept away. You might say to yourself, This is anger, or This is sadness. This simple act of recognition can diminish the intensity of these emotions and create space for acceptance. Journaling is also a beneficial practice. Writing about your feelings allows you to organize them and reflect on your journey. You can jot down memories, express emotions, or even describe moments from your day. There's no right or wrong way to journal; the key is to make it a safe space for your thoughts. Incorporating these mindfulness techniques can gently steer you toward a place of present-moment awareness, offering comfort and a clearer perspective during challenging times.

Acceptance strategies play a crucial role in working through grief. Embracing your emotions rather than pushing them away can foster a sense of inner peace. Recognizing that it's okay to feel pain encourages gentle self-acceptance.

Instead of criticizing yourself for feeling sad or angry, remind yourself that these reactions are natural responses to loss. You might practice self-compassion by treating yourself as you would treat a dear friend in a similar situation. Speak to yourself with kindness and understanding, acknowledging that grief is a personal journey without a right or wrong way to cope.

A crucial aspect of acceptance involves acknowledging that grief doesn't have a timeline. It ebbs and flows, appearing unexpectedly. Allowing yourself to feel whatever comes up can lessen the burden of trying to meet societal expectations of moving on. You might find it helpful to create a ritual around your grief. This could involve lighting a candle in memory of your loved one or visiting a place that was significant to you both. Such acts of remembrance can foster a connection and provide comfort, solidifying your emotions as part of your ongoing relationship with the one you lost.

In your day-to-day life, you can embrace acceptance by incorporating small moments of mindfulness. Practicing gratitude, even for simple aspects of your life, can shift your focus and create a sense of balance. Consider keeping a gratitude journal where you jot down three things each day that you appreciate, even in the shadow of grief. This practice can help you cultivate a more positive outlook while honoring your feelings. Allow these acceptance strategies to lead you toward embracing your emotional reality, giving you the strength to navigate through this profound journey.

5.2   Creating Rituals for Connection and Closure

When someone close to us passes away or when we face deep emotional endings, creating rituals can help form a meaningful bond both with the person we have lost and with ourselves. These rituals act as a bridge, allowing us to honor memories and express feelings that might otherwise remain unspoken. They don't need to be complicated or formal; even simple, heartfelt actions can foster a sense of closeness. For example, lighting a candle in a quiet moment may become a way to call up the presence of a loved one, giving space for reflection. This kind of personal ceremony creates a connection that goes beyond physical absence and offers comfort through intentional remembrance.

Establishing these moments of ritual encourages us to engage with grief in a thoughtful and self-compassionate way. Taking time to gather photos, write letters, or revisit places shared with a loved one can help us process emotions silently and gently. The practice also supports self-awareness, allowing individuals to find their own rhythms for healing. Some may find solace in repetitive acts like planting a tree or creating a memory box, while others might prefer quieter gestures, like a daily breath taken in honor of the departed. By customizing rituals to fit personal preferences and cultural backgrounds, each person crafts a unique space where feelings can be felt fully and without judgment. This process fosters ongoing connection, even as the world continues to turn.

Rituals also serve to mark transitions in grief and healing, providing a sense of grounding when emotions seem overwhelming. They remind us that while the loss might change the shape of our lives, it doesn't erase the bonds once formed. Making time to acknowledge these ties can ease loneliness and isolation, offering a quiet companionship in moments that might otherwise feel empty.

Through ritual, we actively participate in our own journey, honoring both our pain and the presence of love that remains embedded in memory.

Alongside building emotional connections, creating rituals helps bring a sense of closure. Ceremonial acts allow us to say goodbye in ways that words alone often cannot express. For some, this might mean holding a gathering where stories are shared, laughter mingles with tears, and the community comes together. Others may find comfort in solitary practices, such as writing a final letter that is released into the wind or choosing to release objects or symbols that carry significance. These acts externalize complex feelings and provide physical expressions of farewell, making the process tangible and grounded.

Closure, in this sense, is less about ending grief and more about honoring progress and transformation.

A ritual designed to aid healing could include lighting incense or playing music that was meaningful to the person who has passed. Creating a small altar with treasured items, or simply spending time in nature while speaking aloud the feelings inside, can also help unlock emotions. Setting intentions during these moments serves as an anchor, guiding the heart toward acceptance without rushing the process. Rituals give grief a form when words fail, helping us move forward while still carrying our memories gently.

When designing these ceremonial practices, practical steps often help guide the experience without overwhelming it. Choosing a time and place where you feel safe and undisturbed sets a foundation for sincerity and peace. You might select a quiet morning or evening, a spot outdoors, or a cozy corner indoors, where the ambiance supports reflection. Deciding beforehand what elements will be part of the ritual, such as lighting candles, playing meaningful songs, or speaking certain thoughts aloud, gives structure but leaves room for spontaneity. It's also helpful to set a small intention, whether it's to honor a specific memory or to express feelings that have been held close. These straightforward steps turn abstract emotions into something tangible and approachable.

Creating a ritual doesn't have to be a one-time event. Repeating a ritual regularly can build a comforting routine that helps keep the connection alive while supporting ongoing healing. Whether it's lighting a candle every week on an anniversary or writing a journal entry addressed to the lost loved one, these repeated actions become touchstones in the journey through grief. Time molds the meaning of these rituals, deepening their impact gently without demanding sudden resolution. They help shape a new normal, one that embraces loss without losing sight of life.

Remember, the power of ritual lies in its deep personal nature. Trust your instincts when choosing how to mark moments of grief and closure, and don't hesitate to incorporate your own cultural or spiritual traditions. Sometimes blending old ways with new ones can create a space that feels just right for you. Allow room for emotions to come and go without rushing, knowing each act of remembrance is a step toward honoring a relationship that will always live in your heart

A practical tip for those beginning to create personal rituals is to start small. Even a brief moment of silence, a gentle touch to a meaningful object, or speaking a few quiet words can open pathways to healing. As you build these moments into your routine, you give yourself permission to feel, remember, and find a sense of peace that carries through the days.

5.3 Developing a Supportive Routine During Grief

When dealing with loss, daily routines can serve as a steadying force amid feelings of chaos and uncertainty. Having familiar activities to rely on each day creates a sense of order that can be comforting. This could mean waking up and going to bed at the same time, eating regular meals, or setting aside certain times for specific activities. Keeping routines uncomplicated and manageable helps prevent feeling overwhelmed. Even small actions, like taking a short walk or tidying up a space, can establish a rhythm that slowly rebuilds a feeling of normalcy.

Consistency doesn't mean every day has to look the same, but having some predictable parts can provide reassurance. It's okay to adjust routines as you go along—what matters most is that they help you feel a foothold during difficult days. Over time, these small routines accumulate into a foundation that can make larger responsibilities, or emotional struggles feel a little less daunting.

The key is to start with simple, achievable steps and gradually add stability wherever possible, giving yourself permission to take things one day at a time.

Creating a predictable schedule also helps to keep your mind grounded. For example, dedicating specific times in the day to work, rest, or connecting with others can make a noticeable difference. Writing down key parts of your routine can serve as a gentle reminder, especially on days when energy or motivation feels low. Having these routines in place doesn't erase grief but offers a gentle structure to support your healing journey. It's about finding small anchors that remind you of what remains steady, even when feelings are fluctuating widely.

Self-care is essential during grief, but it doesn't always mean big gestures or time-consuming activities. Sometimes, simple acts like drinking enough water, eating nourishing meals, or taking a few deep breaths can provide much-needed relief. Setting aside even a few moments each day to check in with yourself helps maintain a connection to your needs. Mindfulness activities like slow breathing, gentle stretching, or paying close attention to your surroundings can ground you when emotions become overwhelming. These practices don't solve everything, but serve as gentle reminders to care for yourself in a kind and compassionate way.

Incorporating small, intentional activities into your routine can build emotional resilience gradually. For example, journaling thoughts or feelings, listening to calming music, or taking brief walks can all contribute to a sense of stability.

The goal isn't perfection but consistency, creating opportunities for moments of peace and self-awareness. As you develop these habits, they can act as anchors during difficult days, making the emotional ups and downs more manageable.

Remember, even brief moments of self-kindness can accumulate into a stronger foundation for well-being as you move through grief.

Fostering routines that include self-care also remind you that your feelings are valid. When grief feels heavy, it's easy to neglect personal needs, but small acts of kindness toward yourself help reinforce your resilience. Producing a routine that incorporates regular check-ins, quiet time, or gentle movement provides signals to your mind that it is safe to rest and heal. These activities don't have to take up much time or be complicated—they simply serve as touchpoints that reinforce your effort to remain connected with your well-being. Building this into daily life creates gentle pathways toward emotional strength and steadiness over time.

A practical tip is to set a specific time each day dedicated to self-care, no matter what's happening around you. Whether it's five minutes of breathing exercises or enjoying a favorite cozy activity, committing to these moments helps make self-care a consistent habit. Small steps like this can eventually turn into a supportive routine that feels natural and reliable, giving your mind a break when grief becomes heavy. The focus is on nurturing yourself day by day, creating space for healing and resilience to grow gradually amidst the challenges you face.

🌸 Summary of Core Takeaways

1. Mindfulness and breathing ground you when emotions overwhelm.

2. Acceptance allows pain to soften into peace over time.

3. Rituals personalize healing, connecting love and memory.

4. Consistent routines rebuild stability and confidence.

5. Self-care and mindfulness nurture both body and spirit.

Chapter 6
The Role of Therapy and Counseling

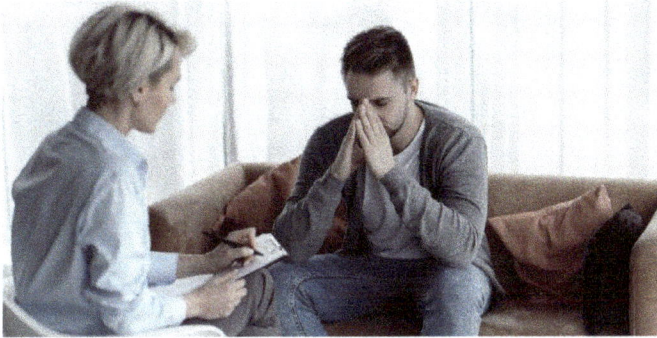

6.1 Choosing the Right Therapeutic Approach for Grief

Grief can make the world feel unsteady, as though the ground you once trusted has shifted beneath your feet. Simple things—like getting dressed, making decisions, or speaking with others—can feel heavy and unfamiliar. In times like these, therapy or counseling can become a safe harbor: a place to pause, breathe, and find your bearings again.

Many people hesitate to seek help because they think they should be able to handle grief alone. They tell themselves, *"I just need more time,"* or *"Others have gone through worse."* But grief isn't a problem to solve—it's a weight that asks to be shared. The right kind of support lightens that weight without demanding that you move faster than your heart is ready for.

Therapy, at its heart, isn't about being analyzed or fixed. It's about being seen. It's a space where you can let your guard down and speak the truth you've been carrying quietly. A good counselor listens not just to your words but to the spaces between them—the sighs, the pauses, the tears you don't want to shed. In that sacred space of listening, something begins to shift: pain starts to loosen its grip, and you begin to feel less alone in your sorrow.

When Words Become Healing

Sometimes, what the heart cannot hold alone begins to heal when spoken aloud. Talk therapy creates that opening. In a session, you might find yourself describing moments you've never shared before—the shock of loss, the guilt of unfinished words, the strange emptiness that lingers after everyone else has gone back to their routines.

The act of putting grief into words is powerful. Each sentence helps untangle emotions that have been twisted together—anger, sadness, guilt, and confusion. Speaking them aloud turns vague, overwhelming pain into something you can look at with gentleness.

A compassionate therapist doesn't rush you toward closure or tell you what you should feel. They walk beside you, reflecting back what you already know deep down: that your grief is valid, your love was real, and your healing will come in its own time. Over weeks or months, these conversations become a quiet rhythm—a meeting between truth and tenderness where you slowly reclaim pieces of yourself you thought were lost.

When the Mind Feels Trapped

Grief doesn't just hurt the heart—it can cloud the mind. Thoughts may loop endlessly, whispering *"What if?"* or *"I should have done more."* These thoughts can grow heavy, feeding guilt or self-blame that keeps the spirit weary.

In gentle, reflective therapy—sometimes called cognitive or insight-based work—the goal is not to erase those thoughts but to bring kindness to them. You might begin to notice when your inner voice turns cruel and learn to meet it with compassion instead of criticism.

A therapist might ask softly, *"What would you say to a friend who felt this way?"* That single question can shift everything. It helps you realize how hard you've been on yourself and invites you to extend the same understanding to your own heart.

Over time, the mind begins to settle. You still remember what happened, but the constant replay of regret begins to fade. The story of your loss doesn't vanish—it transforms from one of self-blame to one of love, courage, and learning.

6.2 Implementing Evidence-Based Interventions (e.g., CBT, EMDR)

Some grief doesn't speak in sentences. It lives in the body, in restlessness, silence, or exhaustion. For these moments, creative or expressive therapies—like art, writing, movement, or music—offer ways to release emotion without needing to explain it.

You might paint with colors that mirror your feelings, write letters you'll never send, or listen to music that lets tears fall without words. These practices aren't about skill or art—they're about expression. They let the heart breathe in a language beyond logic.

In drawing or writing, you may notice patterns: a recurring image, a phrase, or a color that reflects your inner world. Over time, these small creations become markers of healing—a visual map showing how pain is slowly turning into presence, how sorrow is becoming softer.

The Healing Power of Community

Though grief often feels isolating, healing thrives in connection. Group therapy or grief support circles offer a gentle reminder: *you are not the only one walking this road.*

In a group setting, you might sit among strangers who quickly begin to feel like kin. As you listen to others share their stories, you recognize pieces of your own. Someone else's words might bring comfort, or their tears might give you permission to finally release your own.

Community healing isn't about comparing pain; it's about witnessing it together. In these gatherings, there is no need to pretend, no pressure to be strong. Instead, there's understanding, empathy, and the quiet realization that broken hearts still beat in rhythm with one another.

Even outside formal therapy, connection matters. Talking with a trusted friend, joining a faith-based or community group, or volunteering can reawaken a sense of belonging. Grief softens when it meets shared humanity.

When the Weight Becomes Too Heavy

There are times when grief grows too dark to manage alone. You may feel empty for weeks, find no joy in things you once loved, or struggle to get through the day. You may even begin to wonder if healing is possible.

In these moments, reaching out for professional help is an act of profound courage. It's not weakness—it's hope. It's saying, *"I want to live, even if I don't know how right now."*

Therapists are trained to guide you through those darker waters. They can help you find stability, rebuild routines, and remind you that life still holds beauty waiting to be rediscovered. Sometimes medication, mindfulness, or holistic practices become part of the plan; other times, it's simply about having a steady presence walking beside you until your strength returns.

You don't have to reach rock bottom to ask for help. The sooner you open that door, the sooner light begins to seep back in.

6.3   Building a Collaborative Therapist-Client Relationship

The relationship between therapist and client is unlike any other. It's built on trust, patience, and presence. In this space, you don't have to hide your sorrow or defend your emotions. You're free to bring your full, unfiltered self—the grief, the numbness, the anger, the small flickers of hope—and know it will all be met with acceptance.

A skilled therapist doesn't push you out of grief; they walk through it with you. They help you understand that healing isn't the absence of pain, but the gradual rediscovery of life beyond it. Over time, therapy becomes less about talking through loss and more about learning to live with it—integrating it as part of your story rather than an open wound.

The most profound healing often happens quietly. You may not notice it at first—the moments when you laugh without guilt, when you wake with a little more energy, or when you realize a memory no longer hurts quite as sharply. That's therapy's subtle power: helping you rediscover the capacity for life that grief had hidden away.

A Closing Reflection

Therapy is not a finish line; it's a journey alongside your grief. It offers understanding, structure, and compassion when you have none left to give yourself. Whether you choose one-on-one counseling, a creative outlet, or a group circle, each step toward support is a declaration that your healing matters.

There's no shame in seeking guidance. There is strength in saying, *"I can't do this alone."* Because none of us are meant to. Healing often begins the moment we allow someone else to hold our story with us, even for a little while.

And in time, as you speak, create, and connect, you may discover something unexpected: grief no longer defines you. It has become a chapter of your life, yes—but one that shaped your empathy, deepened your spirit, and reminded you that love, even through loss, endures.

🌸 Summary of Core Takeaways

1. **Fit first:** Choose therapy that matches your needs, beliefs, and type of loss.
2. **CBT clarifies and re-engages; EMDR calms traumatic hotspots.**
3. **Evidence-based + compassionate alliance = safety and progress.**
4. **Healing isn't linear; track and adjust with your therapist.**
5. **Trust, transparency, and flexible, client-led goals make therapy work.**

Chapter 7
Building Resilience and Emotional Strength

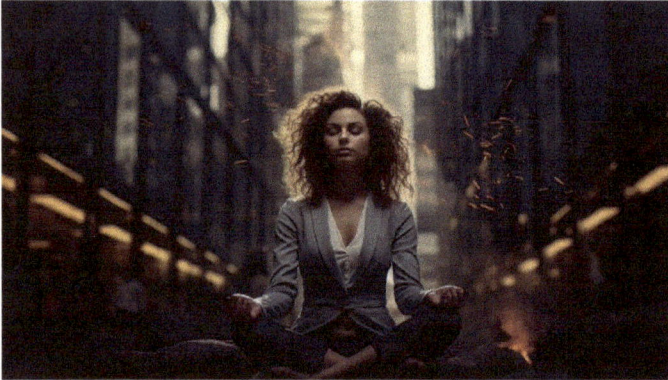

7.1   Techniques for Enhancing Emotional Regulation

Emotional regulation plays a significant role in building resilience, especially during the challenging times of grief. Grieving can bring intense feelings such as sadness, anger, and confusion, making it essential to learn how to manage these emotions effectively. When you can regulate your emotions, you create a more stable environment for yourself, which helps in navigating the ups and downs of loss.

Emotional regulation doesn't mean suppressing your feelings; instead, it involves understanding and responding to them in healthy ways. This ability allows you to process your emotions rather than be overwhelmed by them. It helps you to find a balance between feeling your grief and carrying on with daily activities.

Developing this skill opens the door to healing, allowing you to honor your feelings while also taking steps toward recovery. By enhancing your emotional regulation, you create a solid foundation that supports you throughout your grieving journey. Mindfulness is one effective technique to enhance emotional regulation.

By focusing on the present moment without judgment, you can better understand your emotions as they arise. This practice helps you to cultivate awareness of your feelings, allowing you to observe them without becoming consumed. You can start with simple exercises, such as spending a few minutes each day focusing on your breath, noticing your surroundings, or observing your thoughts without reacting.

This can create space between your emotions and your responses, giving you time to choose how to react rather than reacting impulsively. Deep breathing is another practical method that can quickly calm the mind and body when you're feeling overwhelmed. Taking slow, deep breaths helps to activate the body's relaxation response, lowering stress levels and helping you feel more centered.

To practice, try inhaling deeply through your nose for a count of four, holding your breath for a count of four, and then exhaling slowly through your mouth for another count of four. Repeat this several times and notice how it helps you manage your emotions more effectively. Cognitive reframing is a technique that involves changing the way you perceive a situation or emotion.

When you experience negative thoughts during your grieving process, take a moment to challenge them. Ask yourself if there's another way to view your situation that is more positive or less distressing. For example, instead of thinking, "I will always be sad," you can reframe your thought to, "I am allowed to feel sad, but I can also find joy in my memories.

" This shift can help you regain a sense of control over your emotional responses and ultimately facilitate your healing process. Combining these techniques regularly can create a powerful approach to emotional regulation. By establishing a routine that incorporates mindfulness, deep breathing, and cognitive reframing, you not only equip yourself with tools for managing grief but also build resilience for the future.

Make the commitment to practice these techniques daily, even in small ways, so they become integrated into your life. By doing so, you will enhance your emotional well-being and find greater ease in navigating the complexities of grief.

7.2 Developing Self-Compassion and Patience

Self-compassion is often overlooked when we face the deep pain of grief, but it plays a crucial role in healing. When you lose someone dear, your emotions can feel overwhelming and unmanageable, making it easy to become your own harshest critic. Instead of offering yourself kindness, you might replay mistakes, blame yourself, or compare your grief to others'.

This often deepens the pain and creates barriers to recovery. Developing self- compassion means treating yourself with the same kindness and understanding you would offer a close friend in distress. It lays the groundwork for resilience by helping you accept your feelings without judgment, which is a necessary step toward emotional recovery.

At the core of self-compassion is acknowledging that grief is a natural, human experience. It's not a sign of weakness to feel lost or vulnerable; rather, it's a part of what makes us human. When you allow yourself to think without criticism, you create space for healing to begin.

This does not mean ignoring your pain or pushing it away; it means recognizing your experience and responding with patience and gentleness. Some find it helpful to remind themselves that no one moves through grief in a straight line or according to a set timeline. Everyone's journey is different, and offering yourself grace throughout this time strengthens your ability to cope with the challenges ahead.

Patience becomes a vital companion when dealing with grief. Healing often unfolds slowly, and it doesn't follow a predictable path. There will be moments when progress feels steady and others when it seems as though you are stuck or even moving backward.

This can be frustrating, but patience helps ease the tension that comes from wanting to hurry the process. Recognizing that healing is gradual reduces the pressure to "get over" your loss quickly. It invites the understanding that setbacks are part of growth, not signs of failure.

Over time, patience nurtures a softer way of relating to yourself, one that embraces imperfection and accepts the unpredictability of grief. Alongside patience, cultivating self-acceptance means allowing yourself to feel whatever arises without criticism. This can be difficult during grief because the emotions involved—sadness, anger, confusion—may seem overwhelming or even frightening.

Yet accepting these feelings as normal and temporary helps avoid the extra burden of self-judgment. When you accept what you're experiencing, you build a foundation for healing that honors your pace and your process. Remind yourself that feeling vulnerable does not make you less strong.

It shows that you are human, and in that space of acceptance, there is room for gentle growth and renewal. One practical way to develop patience and self- acceptance is by focusing on small daily moments instead of the entire journey. Celebrate simple victories, like allowing yourself a moment of rest or expressing your emotions without shame.

These tiny acts of kindness to yourself accumulate and create a shift in how you view your grief. Patience and self-compassion are not about rushing to feel better; they are about being with yourself as you heal, no matter how long it takes.

7.3 Leveraging Support Networks and Community Resources

When going through a time of loss, it can feel overwhelming to face each day alone. Support networks, whether family, friends, or community groups, play a crucial role in helping navigate these tough moments. They offer a comforting presence, allowing the grieving person to share feelings without fear of judgment. Having people who listen and understand can lessen feelings of loneliness and remind someone they are not alone in their pain. Building and learning about these connections can provide a foundation of stability during uncertain times. Recognizing the value of support networks encourages individuals to seek out and accept help, making the healing process less lonely and more manageable.

Support networks do more than just listen; they also provide practical assistance. This might include helping with daily chores, running errands, or offering transportation to appointments. Such help can ease the burden of daily responsibilities, freeing up more emotional energy for processing grief.

Support networks often serve as a source of encouragement, reminding those who mourn that healing takes time and that they can face each new day. Having a group of reliable people to turn to can prevent feelings of despair from taking over completely. This shared strength can foster resilience and create a safe space for expressing a wide range of emotions, from sadness to hope.

Understanding the importance of these networks encourages people to actively cultivate relationships before they're needed the most. Small acts of reaching out, maintaining contact, and offering support in return can strengthen bonds over time. When grief hits, these established connections become a natural source of comfort.

Sometimes, simply knowing there is someone to call or visit can make a big difference. The support can extend beyond friends and family to include spiritual leaders, colleagues, or members of local support groups. Recognizing the importance of a supportive environment helps individuals build a safety net before experiencing loss, making the journey through grief less isolation-filled and more connected.

Many communities offer a variety of resources designed to support those who are grieving. Local churches, community centers, and nonprofits often run groups or programs specifically for people dealing with loss. These groups provide a space to share experiences and gain insights from others who understand what it feels like.

Sometimes, there are free or low-cost counseling services provided by community organizations that can help process intense emotions. Additionally, community resource directories—available online or at local centers—list services such as crisis hotlines, volunteer visitors, or grief support classes.

Knowing where to look can make it easier to find help when feeling overwhelmed or unsure of what steps to take next.

Accessing practical assistance through community resources can also ease the day-to-day challenges that come with grief. For example, some organizations offer rides to medical appointments, help with household chores, or provide meals. These kinds of support can temporarily lift burdens, allowing individuals to focus more on their emotional well-being.

Many communities also hold workshops on coping skills, mindfulness, or self-care, giving people useful tools for managing grief. Getting involved in these programs or reaching out for help can create a sense of connection and reassurance, demonstrating that support is available in many forms. It's often helpful to talk with a social worker, counselor, or community center staff to navigate available options.

Starting with small steps can open doors to a wider network of assistance. Asking trusted friends or family members for recommendations, or calling local organizations directly, can quickly connect individuals with the help they need. Even just visiting a support group for grief can provide guidance and companionship.

Many programs are designed to be welcoming and non-judgmental, creating a sense of community and shared understanding. Remember, seeking help is a sign of strength and readiness to heal. Keeping informed about available resources ensures that support is accessible when needed most, offering comfort and practical aid throughout the grieving process.

🌸 Summary of Core Takeaways

1. Emotional regulation is the backbone of resilience—feel fully, respond wisely.

2. Mindfulness, deep breathing, and cognitive reframing cultivate calm awareness.

3. Self-compassion and patience dismantle self-criticism and invite gentleness.

4. Healing is nonlinear—celebrate small steps and forgive delays.

5. Support networks and community resources turn solitude into solidarity.

6. Asking for help and staying connected are acts of resilience, not weakness.

Chapter 8
Expressive Arts and Creative Outlets in Healing

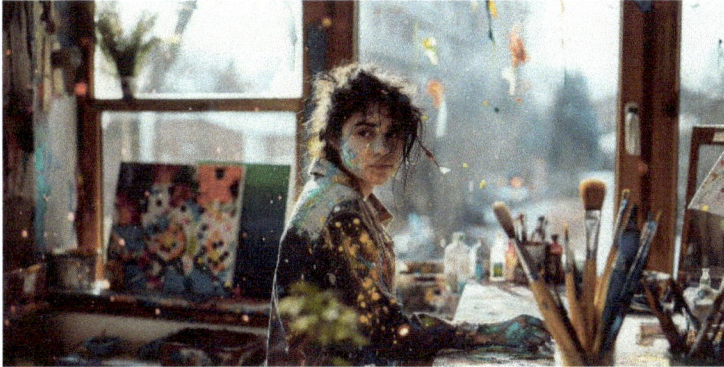

8.1 Using Art, Music, and Writing to Process Grief

Engaging in visual arts, music, and writing can be a powerful way to express emotions and foster healing during the grieving process. These creative outlets provide individuals with a safe space to explore their feelings, allowing for deeper emotional understanding and release. Through painting, drawing, or sculpting, one can convey feelings that may be too complex or painful to articulate in words.

The tactile experience of creating art can also ground individuals, helping them reconnect with their bodies and emotions. Music offers another avenue for emotional expression. Listening to favorite songs or composing original music can evoke memories and feelings that are often locked away in sorrow.

Strumming a guitar or playing a piano can be an outlet for sadness or even a celebration of the loved one's life. Writing, whether through journaling or poetry, can help in processing thoughts and emotions, giving voice to grief that feels too overwhelming to speak aloud. Incorporating creative activities into the grieving process can be both practical and therapeutic.

Setting aside specific times in your routine for art, music, or writing can create a consistent outlet for feelings. For instance, a weekly painting session can become a cherished ritual. You might start by choosing a comfortable space and gathering materials such as paints, brushes, or canvas.

As you create, focus on what you are feeling in that moment. It's about the process, not the outcome. Similarly, consider dedicating time to playing music or listening to tracks that resonate with your emotions.

Create a playlist that speaks to your journey through grief. When words fail, music can fill that void, giving you comfort and a sense of companionship. Writing a letter to the deceased can be another effective method.

Expressing everything you wish you could have said can provide a sense of closure and connection, almost as if you're carrying on a conversation. Even simple journaling, where you jot down thoughts about your day or your feelings, can be incredibly grounding. Reflecting on your creative journey can also deepen your understanding of your grief.

Keep your artwork, music, and writings as a record of your emotional landscape. As time passes, revisiting these creations can reveal how much you have grown and how your feelings have evolved. It's important to remember that there is no right or wrong way to grieve or to express that grief.

Each person's experience is unique. Embracing the creative process can be a gentle reminder that healing is not linear. It is a journey filled with ups and downs.

Allow yourself the grace to create without judgment and know that each piece you produce is part of your personal healing journey. To help you begin, gather your materials and set a time this week to focus entirely on your chosen art form. Whether it's writing, painting, or playing music, immerse yourself in the process and see where your emotions take you.

8.2 Incorporating Creative Practices into Daily Life

Incorporating creative practices into daily life doesn't require hours of free time or special skills. Simple activities like doodling while on a phone call, writing brief reflections in a journal, or even arranging flowers can become natural parts of a routine. Starting small helps make these practices sustainable and comfortable, especially during times when emotions feel overwhelming.

For instance, dedicating just five minutes each morning to sketch or write can gradually become a comforting ritual that provides relief and clarity. The key is consistency; even fleeting moments of creative expression can act as gentle anchors during challenging days. Over time, these small acts build a sense of normalcy and allow healing to unfold gradually without adding stress or pressure.

To make creativity a regular part of life, find ways to connect it with daily activities. Cooking can turn into a chance for artistic expression by trying new recipes or plating food beautifully. Gardening offers a tactile outlet that connects you with nature and allows for moments of quiet reflection.

Using music as a background during chores or work can influence your mood gently and provide an emotional release. Setting aside a specific time each day, like a few minutes before bed or during a lunch break, helps create a routine. Remember, the goal isn't perfection but allowing yourself the freedom to express feelings in ways that feel natural.

Small, consistent acts of creativity reinforce healing and provide ongoing comfort during tough times. Creating a space that's welcoming and calming makes a big difference when practicing creativity regularly. Choose a quiet corner or a dedicated spot where you can leave your supplies out without worry or clutter.

Filling this area with meaningful objects, like family photos, stones, or favorite books, can inspire calm and remind you of support. Soft lighting, comfortable seating, and minimal distractions help foster a sense of safety, so expressing emotions through art feels less intimidating. Setting gentle intentions for your creative times, such as focusing on feelings rather than results, removes pressure and invites a relaxed, open attitude.

Over time, this nurturing environment nurtures trust in your own expression and creates a space where healing can happen naturally. Making creativity part of everyday life also involves being kind to yourself and embracing imperfection. It's helpful to keep supplies accessible and easy to use, so you're more likely to turn to them when needed.

Incorporate soothing sounds or nature elements, like birdsong or a small indoor fountain, to deepen the sense of peace. Encouraging gentle routines—such as lighting a candle before starting or playing soft music—sets a calming tone. Remember, maintaining an environment that feels safe and inviting shows your commitment to your healing journey, reminding you that in creativity, there is no right or wrong— only honest expression.

Another practical tip is to set gentle intentions for your creative time, such as focusing on how it makes you feel rather than what the outcome looks like. This shift in perspective helps reduce self-criticism and encourages ongoing participation. Keeping a few favorite supplies within reach—like colored pencils, a small sketchbook, or calming coloring pages removes barriers to starting.

An environment that feels both safe and inspiring nurtures your ongoing process of healing, providing a space where emotions can surface naturally and be expressed freely.

🌸 Summary of Core Takeaways

1. Art, music, and writing turn emotion into expression and clarity.
2. The process matters more than the product—creation itself heals.
3. Daily creative habits restore rhythm and balance to emotional life.
4. Safe, inspiring environments encourage honesty and release.
5. Gentle intentions and self-kindness deepen trust in the healing journey.

Chapter 9
Navigating Difficult Emotions and Setbacks

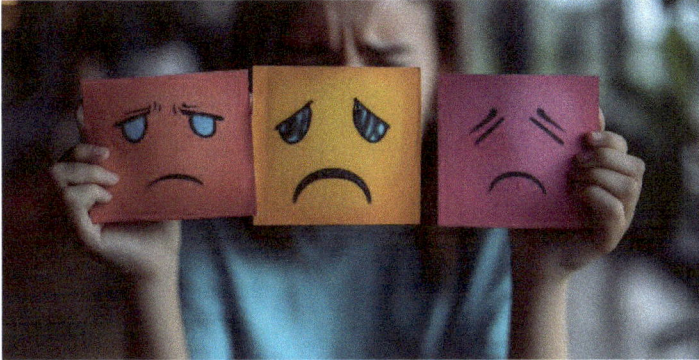

9.1   Identifying and Validating Complex Emotions

Grief is not a simple emotion, but a complex spectrum that can feel overwhelming. It encompasses a variety of feelings such as sadness, anger, confusion, and guilt. Understanding these emotions is crucial for anyone navigating the difficulties of loss.

Often, people think of grief as just sadness, which can lead to misunderstanding the full experience. For example, you may feel angry toward the person who passed away for leaving you or even toward yourself for things you wish you could have done differently. Recognizing that it's normal to have these differing feelings helps in fostering both self-love and empathy from others.

Complex emotions like regret might also surface, often tied to unresolved issues or things left unsaid. As someone grieving, acknowledging these feelings can be challenging, and it's common to feel isolated. Many might even mask their grief with a façade of normalcy, believing that the world expects them to continue as if nothing has changed.

Yet, understanding that this intricate tapestry of emotions is part of the grief process can help ease the burden. Feeling a mix of emotions does not mean you are moving backward in your healing journey; rather, it is a sign that you are engaging with your feelings. Recognizing and affirming your emotions is crucial for healing.

One effective method is to keep a grief journal. Writing about your feelings allows you to process them, providing an outlet for emotions that may otherwise feel trapped inside you. Describe your feelings in detail, whether you're feeling good one day or overwhelmed the next.

Naming these emotions helps in understanding them better, which is the first step toward emotional validation. This practice creates a safe space to explore and confront every ripple of feeling you may experience, validating that these emotions are real and important. You might also find it helpful to share your emotions with someone you trust.

This could be a friend, family member, or therapist who understands grief. Simply expressing how you feel can lead to a sense of relief and connection. Remember that there's no timeline for grief, nor is there a right way to feel.

By talking about your complex emotions or even just sitting in silence with someone who understands, you honor your unique experience. Often, interactions like these become a grounding force, reminding you that you are not alone in your journey. Engaging in creative arts can also serve as a powerful tool for expression.

Drawing, painting, or playing music can help articulate emotions that feel too deep for words. These activities open doors to express feelings creatively, forging a path toward healing. By coming to terms with complex emotions through various methods, you foster not just awareness but also self-compassion, setting the foundation for a healthier healing process.

9.2 Strategies for Managing Guilt, Anger, and Regret

When dealing with grief, guilt, anger, and regret often surface as powerful emotions that can feel overwhelming. The first step in managing these feelings is to acknowledge them without judgment. It's natural to want to push away uncomfortable emotions, but allowing yourself to notice them, whether through writing, talking, or simply sitting with them, helps prevent them from building up inside.

Recognizing these feelings means noticing when they arise and naming them clearly, which gives you a chance to respond calmly instead of being consumed by them. A useful way to process intense emotions is to set small, manageable time limits around them. For example, dedicate ten or fifteen minutes to reflect on what's behind your anger or guilt, then gently bring your focus back to something soothing or grounding.

This approach helps prevent feelings from spiraling and allows you to return to your day without carrying unbearable weight. Practicing deep breathing or meditation during these moments can also create space between you and the emotion, making it feel less immediate and less threatening. It is also helpful to write down your thoughts and feelings as they occur.

Journaling can provide a safe place to express guilt, anger, or regret without fear of misunderstanding or judgment. Sometimes, putting these emotions into words makes them easier to understand and manage. Over time, looking back at your writing can reveal patterns or triggers that you might not have seen before, helping you approach those feelings more kindly and with better tools in the future.

Another key strategy involves setting boundaries with yourself and others around these emotions. It's okay to say no to conversations that dig too deeply when you're not ready or to limit contact with people who intensify your feelings of guilt or anger. Recognizing when a feeling is becoming too much and stepping back from it temporarily is a form of self-compassion.

Avoiding isolation can also ease the burden of heavy emotions. While it's essential to sit with your feelings, reaching out to trusted friends, family, or a counselor can provide emotional support. Sometimes, just knowing that someone else acknowledges your pain can reduce feelings of shame or anger and make processing easier.

Remember, these feelings don't have to be battled alone. One way to soften the impact of guilt, anger, and regret is to reframe how you view these emotions. Instead of seeing them as signs of weakness or failure, consider them as natural responses that highlight your deep care or the significance of your loss.

Viewing these feelings as a form of love or attachment can change their meaning and reduce self-criticism. For example, anger toward a situation or person may reflect the pain of unmet expectations or the helplessness felt during loss. Developing self-compassion is essential in this reframing process.

Talk to yourself as you would to a close friend who is hurting. Remind yourself that making mistakes, feeling angry, or wishing things could have gone differently does not make you a bad person. Compassion creates space for healing and allows you to accept feelings rather than fight against them.

When regret arises, acknowledge that hindsight often brings clarity that wasn't available at the time, and that everyone acts with the information they have in the moment. Mindfulness practices can also promote emotional resilience. Focusing on the present moment prevents you from ruminating on what could have been or fueling anger about the past.

Simple mindfulness exercises, such as paying attention to your breath or observing your surroundings without judgment, help create calm and make it easier to face difficult emotions calmly. Over time, this steadiness allows you to respond to feelings with understanding rather than reacting impulsively. Another way to build resilience is by creating small rituals that honor your feelings and your loss.

Light a candle, plant a tree, or write a letter to your loved one as a way to express guilt, anger, or regret safely. These actions can transform intense emotions into something tangible and meaningful, giving you a sense of control and purpose in a confusing time. They also serve as reminders that your feelings are a part of your journey, not something to push away.

Sharing your experience with others who have faced loss can offer comfort and new perspectives. Hearing how others cope with guilt and regret may help you see that you are not alone in your feelings. It can also open up space for forgiveness, both toward yourself and those involved in your grief story.

Compassion from others often encourages greater self-compassion and resilience, helping you to move forward with greater kindness toward your emotional experience. One practical tip to keep in mind is to remind yourself to breathe deeply whenever strong emotions arise. Taking a few slow, intentional breaths can interrupt intense feelings and bring you back to a place of calm reflection.

This small action anchors you in the moment and creates an opportunity to choose how to respond rather than reacting out of overwhelm.

9.3 Planning for and Responding to Sudden Grief Triggers

Grief triggers can catch you off guard because they often come from familiar places or moments you didn't expect. A song, a scent, a photograph, or even a casual comment can suddenly stir intense feelings. Recognizing that these triggers are a natural part of the healing process helps you avoid feeling overwhelmed when they appear.

Mentally preparing involves accepting that they exist and knowing they are temporary, even if they feel overwhelming. You can try to think of triggers as signals indicating you are processing your feelings, not signs that your grief is returning or worsening. Building awareness about what these triggers might be allows you to face them with a bit more resilience when they show up unexpectedly.

Keeping a small journal of recurring triggers can help identify patterns and prepare you better for future encounters. Preparing yourself mentally also includes developing a mindset that there is no perfect way to handle surprises related to grief. Instead, aim for flexibility and self-compassion.

When you know certain times, places, or activities are more likely to stir emotions, plan around them when possible. For example, if an anniversary or holiday is approaching that might bring up sadness, think about how you'll respond beforehand. Visualizing peaceful responses or reminding yourself that it's okay to feel upset can help reduce the shock if those moments arrive unannounced.

Taking small steps, like setting aside a quiet space or having a calming activity ready, can make an unexpected trigger easier to manage. Over time, these mental preparations build confidence, helping you handle surprises with composure instead of panic or frustration. When a sudden trigger catches you off guard, taking a moment to breathe deeply often helps before reacting.

A few slow breaths can slow your heart rate and give you a moment to collect yourself. If you're in a public place or around others, discreetly grounding yourself by noticing your surroundings can be calming. Reminding yourself that it's okay to feel emotional at times like these is key; it removes some of the pressure to suppress your feelings.

Redirecting your focus toward something comforting, like a picture of someone you loved or a calming phrase, can shift your attention away from distressing thoughts. Allowing yourself to feel emotions without judgment helps prevent them from becoming overwhelming. If possible, giving yourself permission to step away briefly can prevent distress from escalating.

Small acts like taking a walk, finding a quiet corner, or closing your eyes for a moment can give you the space to regain composure. Creating a plan for these situations also involves having practical tools on hand before you face triggers. Carrying a small object that brings comfort, such as a jewelry charm or a smooth stone, can serve as a tactile reminder of stability.

Listening to a favorite calming song or having a list of supportive words written down can provide quick comfort. Practicing mindfulness exercises regularly strengthens your ability to return to a calm state during stressful moments. Building a network of trusted people you can reach out to when triggered can make a big difference.

Sharing your feelings with someone who understands and respects your process offers reassurance and guidance. Remember, the goal isn't to eliminate grief but to find manageable ways to navigate its reactions when surprises happen. Thinking ahead about what tools and strategies work best for you will make a significant difference when unexpected triggers occur.

Sometimes, simply acknowledging that you are feeling overwhelmed and giving yourself permission to have that moment helps break the cycle of panic or sadness. Keep reminding yourself that experiencing strong feelings during triggers is normal, and it signals ongoing processing rather than regression. Building these responses into your daily routine, perhaps through gentle reminders or calming rituals, prepares you better for the unexpected.

With practice, you'll notice that handling sudden grief triggers becomes less daunting and more about managing your response with patience and understanding.

🌸 Summary of Core Takeaways

1. **Name your emotions** — acknowledgment disarms their intensity.

2. **Journal, share, and express creatively** — clarity grows through expression.

3. **Reframe guilt and anger** as signs of deep love, not weakness.

4. **Set boundaries** — protect your healing pace and emotional space.

5. **Plan for triggers** — prepare soothing tools, supportive people, and rituals.

6. **Breathe, ground, and return** — calm begins with one conscious breath.

7. **Remember:** Every wave you face shows that your heart is still capable of love.

Chapter 10
Rebuilding Identity and Purpose Post-Loss

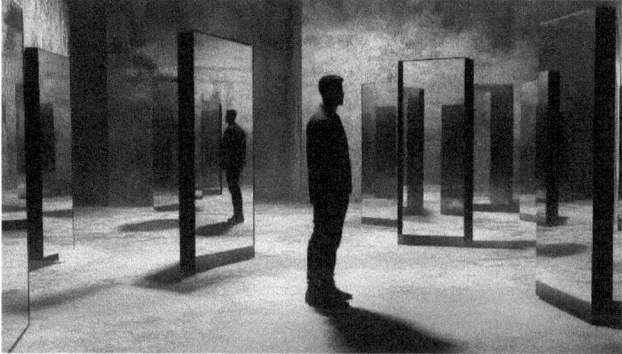

10.1 Redefining Self-Identity After Loss

Experiencing loss can profoundly impact our sense of self. When a loved one passes away, the emotional wound it creates can leave us feeling unmoored, challenging how we perceive our identity. Many people struggle to reconcile their former selves with the new reality they face.

Acknowledging this shift is essential; our identity isn't static but rather a fluid constructr545454 that can change over time. Recognizing feelings of grief and confusion is the first step in navigating this transformation. The journey of redefining oneself after loss is often marked by a complex mix of grief, reflection, and growth.

It's vital to realize that this phase of life can lead to emerging strengths and insights about who we are. By accepting that our identity can evolve, we open the door to rediscovering our passions, values, and sense of purpose that may have shifted in light of our loss. This acknowledgment can bring a certain relief, as it shifts the focus from trying to restore the past to embracing a new way of being.

After recognizing the changing nature of identity, it becomes essential to develop practical strategies that aid in the redefinition of self-perception. One approach is to reflect on the impact of the loss and how it has shaped current feelings and thoughts. Journaling can serve as a valuable tool for exploration, allowing an individual to articulate emotions and experiences that arise in the wake of their loss.

Writing about memories, dreams for the future, and changes in personal beliefs may illuminate the path forward. Another strategy involves connecting with others who understand the experience of loss. Support groups, whether in-person or online, can provide a comforting space to share struggles and triumphs.

Hearing different narratives can inspire new perspectives and ways of thinking. Conversations with trusted friends or family members can also foster deeper discussions that might help in reshaping personal identity. In addition to reflection and support, introducing new activities into one's life can be beneficial.

Engaging in hobbies, volunteering, or pursuing education can bring fresh experiences and opportunities for growth. These activities can not only distract from the pain but also spark joy and connection to life, allowing for the reconstruction of a meaningful narrative. Seeking out activities that resonate with personal interests and values is key; they can act as steppingstones in reclaiming and redefining identity amidst loss.

Finally, embracing the idea that it's okay to feel joy while grieving is a significant step in the journey. Life encompasses a spectrum of emotions, and finding moments of happiness does not diminish the love or memories of the loss. Allowing oneself to find joy creates space for a more integrated self, where loss and new experiences coexist harmoniously.

Understanding that redefining one's identity is an ongoing process can empower individuals to approach life with compassion, curiosity, and an open heart. Establishing a new narrative can take time and patience, but small, deliberate actions can foster healing and growth. Taking purposeful moments to reflect, connect, and engage in life can lead to the development of a renewed self, offering hope for what lies ahead.

10.2 Setting New Goals and Finding Meaning

After experiencing loss, setting new goals can be a way to gently guide yourself forward during a time when everything might feel uncertain or broken. Goals don't have to be large or overwhelming; in fact, starting with realistic, reachable objectives can provide small moments of success that rebuild confidence and offer a sense of control. These goals could be as simple as establishing a daily routine, committing to a short walk, or reaching out to a friend regularly.

By focusing on achievable steps, you create a foundation for healing that acknowledges your current emotions without pushing you too far too fast. This approach encourages gradual personal growth, reminding you that progress isn't about speed but about nurturing yourself patiently. Choosing meaningful goals means thinking about what truly matters to you right now, instead of what might have seemed important before your loss.

Healing often involves more than just moving on—it includes finding ways to honor your feelings and the people you've lost. Setting goals that reflect your current needs and values helps you reconnect with your inner self and offers a clear direction, even when life feels uncertain. Whether it's learning something new, practicing self-care, or volunteering in a way that feels right, these goals support both emotional recovery and a renewed sense of purpose.

They help rebuild the parts of your life that feel empty, offering a path out of pain toward something hopeful and meaningful. When grief has taken center stage, it can be hard to remember what brings you joy or what you stood for before the loss. Taking time to reflect on your core values, those deep beliefs that guide your decisions and define who you are, can provide clarity in the midst of emotional chaos.

These values might be kindness, honesty, creativity, or connection, and recognizing them helps you understand what gives your life meaning beyond the loss you've endured. Looking back on moments when you felt truly alive or proud can highlight passions or interests that still hold significance. This self-discovery is not about erasing grief but about integrating it into a fuller picture of who you are and where you want to go next.

Passions often provide a sense of purpose that can keep you grounded during difficult times. Rediscovering activities that bring you comfort or excitement— even if they feel distant at first—can reignite a spark inside. Whether it's gardening, writing, music, or helping others, these pursuits can serve as anchors that connect you to life's ongoing rhythm.

Alongside your values, passions act as powerful motivators for setting new goals that feel authentic and fulfilling. They remind you that your identity doesn't disappear with loss; it evolves. Finding meaning beyond grief doesn't mean forgetting or moving on too quickly. It means allowing your unique strengths and interests to shape a future where healing and hope can grow side by side.

As you navigate these reflections, consider jotting down moments you feel drawn toward or values that seem most important. This process isn't about rushing to answers but about giving yourself gentle permission to explore who you are now. Purpose may look different from before and that's part of the journey.

Embracing this change can help dissolve feelings of confusion or emptiness by offering a clearer sense of direction. One small tip is to focus on one value or passion at a time, exploring how it might inspire a goal or action. This keeps the process manageable and prevents overwhelm, making growth feel attainable rather than intimidating.

🌸 Summary of Core Takeaways

1. **Identity evolves through loss** — grief reshapes who you are, not just what you feel.

2. **Reflection and connection** reveal new aspects of self and purpose.

3. **Joy is not betrayal** — happiness and mourning can coexist harmoniously.

4. **Small, meaningful goals** restore momentum and rebuild confidence.

5. **Rediscovering values and passions** gives direction when life feels aimless.

6. **Healing means integration, not replacement** — carrying love forward into new life.

7. **Gentle curiosity, patience, and compassion** are the foundation of renewal.

Chapter 11
Supporting Others

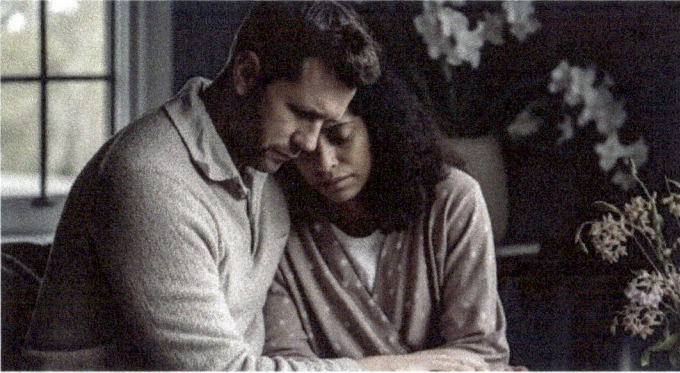

11.1 Effective Communication with the Grieving

Compassion and mindfulness are essential when communicating with someone who is grieving. Grief can leave a person feeling isolated, unsure, and deeply vulnerable. It's crucial to approach conversations with sensitivity and awareness.

A grieving individual may not always express what they need, so tuning into their emotions becomes a vital tool. Establishing a space where they feel safe to share is part of that compassionate approach. Listening without judgment allows them to open up without feeling pressured to conform to social norms about how to grieve.

Consider the nuances of their experience. Each person grieves differently and understanding that their journey is personal can help you offer better support. Being aware of your body language and tone is also important, as these non- verbal cues can communicate care and openness.

Remember, what they may need most is simply for you to be present with them, to acknowledge their pain without trying to fix it. This presence speaks volumes and often offers more comfort than any words could express. Active listening is about fully engaging with the person who is grieving.

This means giving them your complete attention, maintaining eye contact, and not interrupting when they speak. Allow pauses in conversation; silence can sometimes be a necessary part of processing grief. When they do share, they validate their feelings by acknowledging their pain or confusion.

Phrases like "that sounds really hard" can help them feel understood without minimizing their experience. Be cautious of trying to offer solutions, as the grieving may not be looking for advice but simply a compassionate ear. It's essential to avoid common pitfalls, such as comparing their loss to your own experiences or trying to offer silver linings.

Often, statements like "I know how you feel" can come off as dismissive, even if unintentional. Instead, focus on encouraging them to express their feelings and remind them it's okay to feel however they do—sad, angry, lost, or even guilty. Each emotion is valid and a part of their healing journey.

Offering gentle prompts, such as "It's okay to feel that way," can provide necessary reassurance. As you listen, let your responses be guided by their cues; sometimes, simply being by their side can be the most powerful way to communicate support. Keep in mind that grief doesn't follow a linear path.

Be patient and ready to engage in conversations about their loved one, recognizing that reminiscing can both bring joy and increase their sorrow. Acknowledging anniversaries or significant dates can feel daunting but can also open the door for meaningful discussions. Encourage them to share stories, even if it brings tears.

By embracing the depth of their feelings, you help foster an environment of trust where they can feel accepted in their rawness. Remember, your role is to be present, compassionate, and open, ready to stand alongside them as they navigate this difficult journey.

11.2 Providing Practical and Emotional Support

Offering practical support means recognizing what someone needs in their day- to-day life and stepping in to help with those tasks that may feel overwhelming during a time of grief. When a person is mourning, even simple routines like cooking, cleaning, or managing appointments can become difficult to handle. By taking care of these tasks, you relieve some of the burden and create space for them to focus on their emotions and healing.

It's also helpful to be specific in your offers of assistance, such as saying I will bring dinner on Wednesday, or, let me drive you to your doctor's appointment. These clear gestures make it easier for them to accept help without feeling like they are imposing or inconveniencing you. Practical support can also involve helping with things like childcare, running errands, or handling paperwork that often piles up unexpectedly.

Every small act that eases their load can make a meaningful difference. Providing emotional support means being present in a way that honors the grieving person's unique experience. This requires patience and a willingness to listen without rushing to fix their feelings or offer advice.

People who are grieving often need space to share their pain and memories, sometimes over and over again. By simply sitting with them and allowing those emotions to come forward, you show respect for their process. Validation is a key element here acknowledging their feelings without judgment, whether it's sadness, anger, confusion, or relief.

Avoid pushing them to "move on" or suggesting they should feel a certain way. Instead, create an environment where they feel safe to express whatever comes up. Small gestures like maintaining eye contact, nodding, or gentle touches on the hand can communicate empathy without words.

In some cases, silence shared together provides comfort more than any phrase could. Combining practical and emotional support often means balancing doing for someone with being with someone. Practical help solves immediate problems, while emotional support helps them navigate their inner world during a difficult time.

Keeping in touch regularly lets them know you care and are available when they want to reach out. Sometimes, offering both can be as simple as preparing a meal and then sitting together quietly or listening as they talk. If you are unsure what kind of support is needed, it's okay to ask directly, allowing them to guide how you can be most helpful.

Grieving is not a linear experience, and their needs may shift from day to day. By remaining flexible and attentive, you help create a foundation of comfort and reassurance during a period that can otherwise feel isolating. Remember that your presence, whether shown through actions or words, can provide lasting relief and strength in moments of deep vulnerability.

11.3 Recognizing When Professional Help Is Needed

Grief can affect people in many different ways, and not everyone experiences it the same way. Sometimes, signs that indicate a person might need extra help become clear when their emotional reactions are intense or prolonged beyond what they feels is typical. For example, if someone is unable to sleep, constantly feels overwhelmed by sadness, or finds it hard to carry out daily activities, these can be signals that their grief is becoming difficult to manage alone.

Changes in behavior, like withdrawing from friends and family or losing interest in activities they once enjoyed, may also show that support is needed. When feelings of guilt, anger, or despair persist for weeks or months without relief, it might indicate that professional guidance could make a difference. Recognizing these signs early can help prevent grief from turning into deeper mental health issues like depression or anxiety.

Physical symptoms can also provide clues. If someone experiences frequent headaches, stomach issues, or chronic fatigue that seem linked to their emotional state, it shows their body is reacting to their sorrow in a way that may need professional attention. Children and teenagers, in particular, often struggle to express what they are feeling, but they might show their distress through tantrums, withdrawal, or declining grades.

It's important to notice when grief stretches into chronic states of hopelessness or agitation, which could point to the need for counseling. Sometimes, family and friends might find it hard to see these signs clearly, especially if they are trying to give space or comforting words. But understanding these cues can help clarify when a professional's support is necessary to ensure the person gets the help they need to move forward gradually and safely.

Bringing up the idea of seeking help can feel delicate, as grief already involves emotional pain that someone might prefer to handle quietly. It's helpful to approach the conversation with kindness, emphasizing that reaching out for support is a sign of strength, not weakness. Instead of suggesting they are 'broken' or 'not coping' well, focus on how a counselor or therapist can provide tools to manage feelings and navigate the tough days.

Offering to go with them to an appointment, or helping them find a professional, can make the process seem less intimidating. Sometimes, sharing stories of others who benefited from counseling can normalize the idea. The key is to listen without judgment and respect their pace, understanding that grief is a personal journey.

By expressing concern in a gentle way and highlighting the benefits of professional guidance—such as relief, clarity, and coping strategies—you can encourage someone to consider this step without adding to their distress. Simple acts, like providing information about counseling options or suggesting they talk to a trusted health professional, can make a big difference. It's important to avoid pressuring, as pressure can increase feelings of shame or guilt.

Instead, let them know that help is available whenever they feel ready, and that seeking support is a positive act of self-care. Sometimes, framing therapy to better understand their feelings or find peace can resonate more deeply. Remember, patience and understanding go a long way, knowing they have a caring person who respects their space can give someone the confidence to take that initial step toward professional help.

Keep in mind that the goal isn't to force answers but to offer reassurance and options. Sharing resources, like helplines or support groups, can serve as a gentle nudge without overwhelming. Over time, small conversations and consistent kindness can help someone see that seeking help is a healthy choice, especially when they realize they don't have to face their grief alone.

🌸 Summary of Core Takeaways

1. **Listen more than you speak.** Presence comforts more than advice.

2. **Honor individuality.** Every grief story is personal and sacred.

3. **Provide both practical and emotional care.** Love is seen in both action and stillness.

4. **Validate emotions.** "It's okay to feel that way" is powerful medicine.

5. **Discern when to seek professional help.** Wisdom complements compassion.

6. **Support gently and consistently.** Patience sustains the healing journey.

7. **Offer hope without hurry.** Healing unfolds on its own divine timetable.

Chapter 12
Advanced Techniques for Deepening Healing

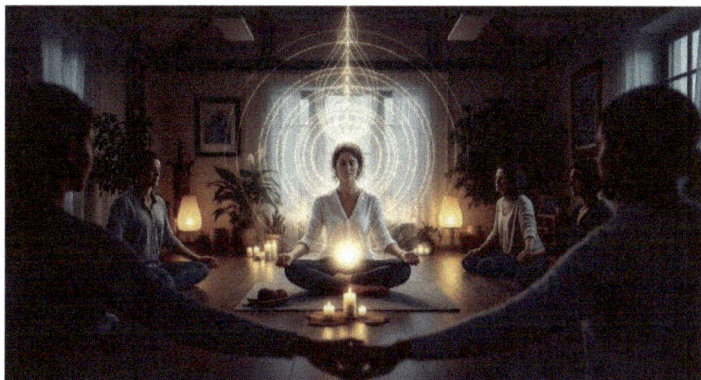

12.1 Integrative Approaches: Combining Mindfulness, Therapy, and Creativity

Mindfulness practices serve as powerful tools for individuals navigating the path of grief. These practices emphasize being present in the moment and accepting feelings   withoutjudgment.   By incorporating mindfulness into therapy, individuals can learn to recognize and confront their emotions rather than avoiding them.

This practice helps foster a sense of awareness around grief, allowing people to explore their feelings in a safe space. Mindfulness encourages individuals to observe their thoughts and feelings, creating a gentle distance from overwhelming emotions. This distance can transform experiencing grief from something all- consuming to something manageable.

Therapeutic settings can introduce mindfulness through various techniques, such as breath awareness, body scanning, or guided imagery. Clients can be encouraged to take a few moments to focus solely on their breath, observing its rhythm and how it feels as they inhale and exhale. This practice not only calms the mind but also creates an opportunity to be present with thoughts and feelings related to grief.

For instance, someone grieving might find themselves feeling waves of sadness. By practicing mindfulness, they can acknowledge this sadness without becoming submerged by it, recognizing it as part of their healing process. Creative expression can be a profound avenue for processing grief.

Art, writing, and music offer unique ways for individuals to connect with their emotions and communicate their experiences. Through these mediums, feelings that are often difficult to articulate can begin to take shape. Engaging in creative activities allows individuals to explore their grief outside the confines of traditional therapeutic dialogues.

For example, someone may choose to paint or draw as a means of illustrating their feelings. Colors and forms can convey emotions that words sometimes fail to express. Writing can also be a powerful tool for reflection and healing.

People can write letters to their lost loved ones, expressing unspoken thoughts or unresolved feelings. This practice can provide clarity and bring peace as individuals articulate their grief on paper. Meanwhile, music can evoke deep emotional responses, whether through listening or creating.

Composing songs or simply selecting melodies that resonate can help individuals honor their grief while connecting with their inner selves. The act of creation, in whatever form, fosters an important connection to emotions and experiences, reinforcing the process of healing. Incorporating these creative outlets into a grieving process not only enhances emotional comprehension but also strengthens one's journey toward acceptance.

People are often surprised by the insights they gain through these methods. One practical tip is to set aside time each week dedicated to creative expression, whether it be writing a journal entry, creating a piece of art, or simply listening to music that reflects their feelings. This practice can help in making the often- intimidating experience of grief feel more manageable.

12.2 Addressing Complicated and Prolonged Grief

Grief is a deeply personal experience, and for some, it extends far beyond the initial waves of sadness and adjustment. Prolonged grief can feel like the pain is frozen in time, preventing healing and making it difficult to engage with life again. This type of grief may come with intense feelings of yearning and an overwhelming sense of loss that stays persistent for months or years.

People struggling with complicated grief often find it harder to accept the reality of the loss or to find meaning in life without the person they lost. This can lead to emotional numbness, social withdrawal, and even problems concentrating or sleeping. Unlike normal grief, which usually eases with time, prolonged grief keeps a person trapped in a cycle of painful memories and avoidance behaviors, complicating the natural healing process.

The impact of this kind of grief extends beyond emotions. It can affect physical health, relationships, and day-to-day functioning. Someone caught in prolonged grief might feel isolated because friends or family expect them to "move on" or feel better with time, which isn't always how grief works.

This disconnect can deepen their sense of loneliness, making it harder to seek support. Often, this grief gets tangled with feelings of guilt, anger, or regret, intensifying the experience. Recognizing prolonged grief can be challenging because it can look like depression or anxiety, but the focus is specifically on the loss and the inability to reassimilate life without the deceased.

Understanding these nuances is key to offering compassion and appropriate help to those struggling to heal. When grief becomes complicated, it's not just about time passed; it involves the way the brain and heart process the loss. Some individuals may have experienced traumatic elements around the death, such as sudden or violent loss, which can compound the grief experience.

Others may have lost someone very close in a relationship where their identity was intertwined deeply with the deceased, making it incredibly difficult to find a sense of self again. The ripple effects might include avoiding reminders of the loved one or obsessively seeking them through memories or interactions with others. These patterns disrupt the emotional work needed to gradually accept loss and form a new normal.

Supporting someone through complicated grief involves patience and recognizing that standard advice like "time heals all wounds" may not hold true. Having clarity about the challenges faced helps in tailoring approaches that address both emotional pain and practical roadblocks to recovery. Advanced therapeutic interventions designed for complicated grief focus on helping individuals gradually engage with their pain in a safe and structured way.

Instead of encouraging avoidance of painful memories, these therapies gently guide people to confront their feelings and memories with support. One such approach includes grief-focused cognitive-behavioral therapy, which helps identify and change unhelpful thoughts connected to the loss. This kind of therapy can help someone reframe feelings of guilt or responsibility, reduce avoidance of reminders, and foster more adaptive coping strategies.

It also often includes techniques that focus on restoring a sense of meaningful connection to life, despite the loss. Another effective method involves exposure therapy, where individuals carefully and gradually face reminders of the loss that they may have been avoiding.

This can include visiting places or looking at photographs that were once painful.

The goal is to reduce fear or distress linked to these reminders, making them less threatening over time. Group therapy can also provide a supportive environment where people recognize they aren't alone in their experience, gaining strength from shared stories and validation. Through connection, those with complicated grief can start to rebuild social bonds and reduce feelings of isolation.

Sometimes, interventions may incorporate mindfulness or acceptance-based strategies to help individuals sit with their emotions without judgment or reaction. These practices can increase tolerance for intense feelings and teach how to observe grief without becoming overwhelmed. Healing from complicated loss involves honoring the pain but not allowing it to dominate life completely.

Therapeutic work often aims to help people find ways to carry their loss forward while gradually re-engaging with their world and relationships. Finding the right approach often requires collaboration between the individual and mental health providers, adjusting treatment based on progress and personal needs. Reminding those who grieve that recovery is not about forgetting but about learning to live fully again can be comforting and empowering.

Sometimes, small shifts in perspective and routine can open doors to healing that once seemed shut tight. A practical tip for those navigating complicated grief is to gently create space for both remembering and moving forward. This might mean intentionally setting aside moments for honoring memories alongside finding something new that brings a sense of purpose or joy.

Grief is rarely a straight path, but with support and the right tools, it becomes possible to find balance amid the pain.

12.3 Using Visualization and Guided Imagery for Closure

Using visualization and guided imagery can be a powerful way to help process grief and find a sense of peace. These methods allow you to create mental images that connect with your feelings, even if words are hard to find. When you picture positive or comforting scenes, your mind begins to shift away from pain and into a space of gentle acceptance.

This doesn't erase the loss but creates a safe mental space where healing can begin. Over time, consistent practice can help you feel less overwhelmed and more connected to feelings of love and remembrance. Visualization is not about pretending the loss never happened; instead, it offers a way to acknowledge your emotions and gradually make peace with them.

Guided imagery takes this a step further by providing stories or scenarios that lead your mind toward comfort and resolution. These techniques are especially useful when feelings of sadness, anger, or guilt become heavy, giving you tools to find moments of calm. They can also help you access courage and resilience, allowing you to carry your memories while moving toward emotional closure.

Using these visual tools can become an integral part of your ongoing healing journey. Practicing visualization and guided imagery creates a gentle space where you're in control. Instead of forcing yourself to 'move on,' you gently invite your mind to explore scenes that support your growth.

These might include imagining yourself wrapping your loved one in a warm light, or sitting by a peaceful river, feeling your feelings wash over you safely. The beauty of these techniques is their flexibility—they can be adapted to meet your emotional needs at any time. When used regularly, they encourage a calmer mind and a heart that's slowly learning to find closure without losing the love that continues to live in your memories.

To get started, it's helpful to find a quiet space where you won't be disturbed. You can sit or lie down comfortably, taking a few slow breaths to settle your body. Remember, there's no 'right' way to do this.

The goal is to create a vivid mental scene that resonates with you, bringing comfort and peace when needed. As your mind learns to picture these gentle images, they become a calming anchor in your daily life, offering reassurance even in difficult moments. With patience, guided imagery can become a gentle companion that helps you move toward emotional closure at your own pace.

Practicing visualization can simply involve closing your eyes and imagining a scene that brings you peace. Examples include watching a loved one's favorite place or imagining a safe, protective light surrounding you. The key is to make the scene as detailed and real as possible, engaging in all your senses.

Feel the warmth of the sun, hear the soft sounds, or smell the familiar scents. This focus on sensory details helps deepen the experience and makes it more effective. Over time, these mental images become familiar sources of comfort, helping your heart gradually find peace with your loss.

Guided exercises are especially helpful when starting out. You might listen to recordings or scripts designed to lead you gently through a calming scene, such as walking through a garden or sitting beside a gentle stream. As you relax into the imagery, words can help direct your focus and encourage your feelings to surface safely.

When completed, take a moment to notice any shifts in your emotions—perhaps a sense of relief or a quiet acceptance. Remember, regular practice makes these visualizations a trusted resource you can turn to whenever grief feels overwhelming. One practical tip is to keep a journal of scenes or images that bring you comfort.

Over time, you may find some images more helpful than others, and your favorites can become go-to representations in moments of distress. Incorporating breathing exercises with visualization deepens the calming effect. For instance, breathe in slowly, imagine filling your lungs with a peaceful light, hold for a moment, then breathe out any tension.

🌿 Summary of Core Takeaways

1. **Integration is healing:** Combining mindfulness, therapy, and creativity harmonizes mind, body, and spirit.

2. **Mindfulness transforms reaction into awareness:** Pain becomes manageable when faced with presence instead of resistance.

3. **Creativity expresses the unspeakable:** Art, writing, and music convert emotion into movement.

4. **Prolonged grief needs gentle, structured care:** Specialized therapy and compassion restore balance and connection.

5. **Visualization brings peace within:** Mental imagery and breath become sacred tools for emotional closure.

6. **Healing doesn't erase love — it reframes it:** You carry the memory not as a wound, but as wisdom.

Chapter 13
Creating a Long-Term Grief Management Plan

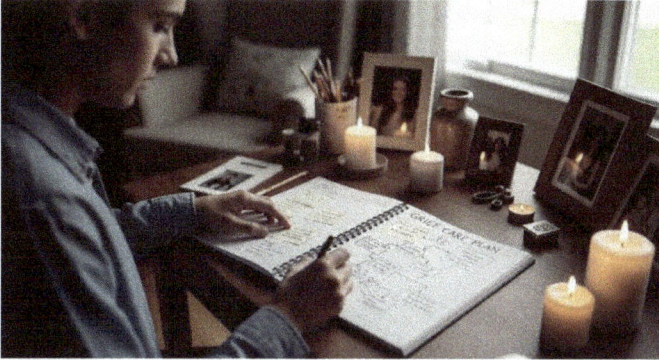

13.1 Developing Personal Rituals and Practices for Ongoing Healing

Personalized rituals play a significant role in the healing process, especially for those dealing with loss. These rituals provide a framework to honor and remember loved ones, creating a sense of ongoing connection that can be profoundly comforting. When someone we care about passes away, it is natural to feel a loss that can sometimes seem overwhelming.

Creating rituals around their memory can help channel grief into something tangible, allowing individuals to navigate their emotions more effectively. Rituals can be anything from lighting a candle on special dates to sharing stories about the person with family and friends. Each act not only acknowledges the loss but also reinforces the bond that continues despite physical absence.

Personalized rituals provide space for reflection and mourning, offering moments of solace amidst the chaos of grief. They are unique to each individual, tailored to reflect the relationship shared with the deceased. For some, participating in an annual Remembrance Day or creating a dedicated space in their home can foster a sense of closeness that transcends everyday life.

By engaging in these practices, individuals can experience their grief in a structured way, leading to a deeper understanding of their emotions and developing a clearer path towards healing. Rituals can also bring communities together, allowing those who share a loss to support one another through shared experiences and remembrance. Designing meaningful rituals requires introspection and personalization, ensuring that they resonate deeply with individual feelings and memories.

Start by considering what aspects of the relationship you wish to honor. This could include favorite activities, shared traditions, or simple gestures that remind you of the loved one. Keeping a journal can be a powerful way to explore these feelings while documenting the rituals as they evolve over time.

You might write letters to your loved one or compose poetry that reflects your emotions. Journaling enables you to express what is often hard to articulate, providing an ongoing emotional release and clarity. Incorporating these practices into daily life can be as simple as establishing small, consistent actions.

This could mean dedicating a few moments each day to reflect on memories or setting aside a specific time each week to engage in a ritual. The key is consistency, as these practices build emotional resilience over time. For example, creating a small memorial space at home with photos and mementos can serve as a daily reminder to pause and reflect.

Similarly, participating in community events that honor those who have passed can create a shared sense of support and understanding. Ultimately, the goal is to cultivate rituals that reinforce connectivity and foster emotional health, enabling individuals to navigate their healing journey in a supportive and enriching manner.

13.2 Monitoring and Adjusting Your Grief Strategies

Creating regular moments to check in with yourself about how you're coping with grief can offer clarity and comfort. Setting aside time each week or even daily— depending on what feels right—helps you stay connected to your emotions and notice any shifts in how you're feeling. This might mean journaling for a few minutes, sitting quietly to reflect, or talking with someone you trust about your experience.

By making these reflections a habit, you allow yourself to track your healing process and recognize if certain strategies you've been using are helping or if they need change. Over time, this routine becomes a way to honor your grief while giving yourself permission to adjust as needed. The benefits of this regular review go beyond just awareness.

It acts as a gentle reminder that grief is not linear, and each day can bring different challenges. You might find that in one week, spending time in nature helps you feel grounded, while another week calls for seeking social support. These reflections provide a space where you are both compassionate and honest with yourself, creating a foundation for healthier grieving rather than suppressing emotions or trying to move on too quickly.

This self-check-in also reduces the risk of becoming overwhelmed by feelings you might not have noticed building up, because by pausing frequently, you're more tuned in to what your heart and mind need now. Grief changes as your life changes, and so should the ways you support yourself through it. When you notice your emotions shifting—whether it's more sadness, anger, or even numbness, it's a signal that your current coping methods might need tweaking.

Flexibility is key; it's okay to try new approaches or step back from things that no longer serve you. For example, if socializing has felt supportive but starts to feel draining, it's perfectly acceptable to scale back and find quieter outlets like creative expression or meditation. Life events such as anniversaries, holidays, or new responsibilities can also stir feelings that call for different strategies, so adapting your grief plan around those moments can ease the process.

Being open to change in your grief management doesn't imply instability or failure—it shows resilience. By tuning into your changing emotional landscape, you create space for growth and healing in ways that are authentic to you. Sometimes this means asking for professional support if grief feels too heavy to carry alone or finding new communities that better match where you are in your journey.

It helps to remind yourself that grief is a personal experience without a fixed timeline, so what works now may shift, and that's based on how your life and feelings evolve. Staying flexible ensures your coping tools continue to provide comfort and strength rather than becoming sources of stress or frustration. One practical tip to support adjusting your grief strategies is to keep a simple journal or note where you record your feelings and what you tried that day or week to cope.

Over time, this collection becomes a personal guide showing patterns and preferences you might not otherwise see. This ongoing awareness creates a framework that can gently guide you toward caring for yourself in ways that respect both your past loss and your present needs.

13.3 Preparing for Anniversaries and Special Dates

Anticipating a significant date after loss can bring a mix of emotions—sadness, nostalgia, or even anxiety. To manage these feelings, it helps to plan both mentally and practically. Think about what might feel most meaningful for you on that day.

If certain activities or memories feel overwhelming, consider setting boundaries or creating a plan to support yourself. Practicing self-compassion is key; allow yourself to feel whatever comes up without judgment. Preparing in advance also means organizing your environment—whether that's setting aside a quiet space for reflection or scheduling activities that bring you comfort.

This proactive approach can reduce feelings of being caught off guard and help create a sense of control during a difficult time. On the practical side, consider marking the date on your calendar, but do so in a way that feels right for you. Some people find it helpful to plan a small gathering with supportive friends or family, while others prefer solitude or private activities.

Gathering items that remind you of your loved one, like photos or keepsakes, can make the day more tangible. It's also useful to have a backup plan if the emotions become too intense—know who to reach out to or what activities might help distract and soothe you. Preparing for the practical aspects of the day, such as notifying close friends or planning some self-care activities, can make a noticeable difference in how you experience these moments.

The goal is to create a balance where you honor your feelings without becoming overwhelmed. Reflecting on what has helped in the past can provide guidance for future anniversaries. Perhaps journaling your feelings or writing a letter to your loved one offers a safe way to process emotions.

You might also consider setting small, achievable goals for the day, such as taking a walk, listening to music, or doing something creative. It's okay to adapt your plans as needed; what worked last year might not feel right now, and that's perfectly acceptable. Remember, the key is to be gentle with yourself and recognize that each anniversary is a personal experience.

Giving yourself permission to feel deeply, and also to take time for what feels meaningful, creates a foundation for navigating these special days with honesty and care. Creating rituals that are tailored to your feelings can turn a difficult day into a more meaningful experience. These can be simple acts, like lighting a candle, playing a favorite song, or visiting a place that held significance for your loved one.

Such activities acknowledge your grief and serve as a way to honor the memory without feeling forced. Personalized rituals are powerful because they give space for genuine emotion and help you feel connected to the person you've lost. Think about what feels authentic for you— whether it's writing a journal, planting a tree, or sharing stories with friends.

The important thing is that these rituals resonate with your feelings and support your healing process. Building support systems around these dates also makes a noticeable difference. Reach out to friends or family members who understand what you're going through, especially those who can listen without judgment.

Sometimes, simply sharing your plan or feelings with someone you trust can provide comfort and reassurance. Consider joining support groups, either locally or online, where you can exchange experiences and coping strategies with others facing similar losses. Creating a small community of understanding individuals can lessen feelings of loneliness and remind you that you're not alone.

Keep in mind that supporting yourself doesn't mean doing everything alone; leaning on others when needed is a sign of strength, not weakness. Incorporating activities that bring you peace and strength into your support plan can reinforce resilience. For example, practicing mindfulness, engaging in gentle exercise, or pursuing a hobby can help channel your emotions constructively.

Maintain flexible expectations for these days, allowing yourself to change plans if needed. Perhaps set a routine that includes a moment of reflection, a comforting activity, or a social connection, whatever feels right. Over time, these personal rituals and support networks can become a vital part of your coping toolkit, making each anniversary a bit more manageable and meaningful.

Remember, the goal is to find avenues that let you honor your feelings while nurturing your well-being.

🌸 Summary of Core Takeaways

1. **Rituals sustain connection** — they transform grief into sacred remembrance.

2. **Reflection and journaling clarify emotions** and trace growth over time.

3. **Flexibility ensures resilience** — grief evolves, so should your healing methods.

4. **Preparation for anniversaries reduces anxiety** and allows intentional remembrance.

5. **Community nurtures endurance** — shared sorrow becomes shared strength.

6. **Everyday peace practices anchor long-term healing.**

Chapter 14
Ethical and Professional Considerations in Grief Support

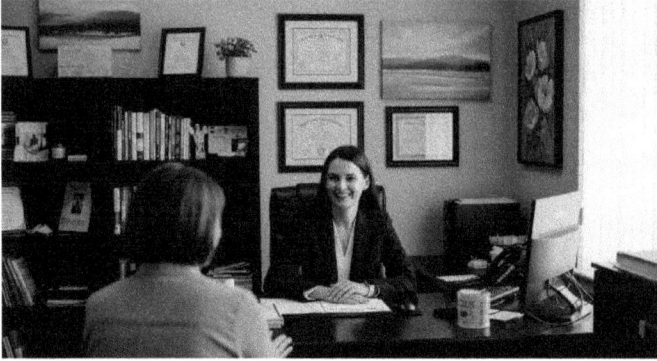

14.1 Maintaining Boundaries and Confidentiality

Establishing and maintaining professional boundaries is crucial for creating a safe space for grieving individuals. These boundaries help define the relationship between the supporter and the person in grief, ensuring that the interaction remains respectful and beneficial. Professionals should communicate clearly about their role and what support they can provide.

This includes explaining the limits of emotional involvement and the necessity of respecting both parties' feelings. Boundaries should also encompass the time spent together and the setting of discussions, aiming for a controlled environment where clients feel comfortable but not overwhelmed. Additionally, setting boundaries helps in preventing dependency.

It is essential for grieving individuals to feel empowered to manage their emotions independently while being supported. Encourage them to seek help, but also remind them that their healing journey is theirs to navigate. This balance fosters resilience and encourages personal growth.

Professionals must remain alert to their own feelings and limits, as the nature of grief can deeply impact those providing support. Staying aware helps in adjusting boundaries if needed. Confidentiality is a cornerstone of building trust with grieving individuals.

Ensuring that personal information shared during supportive conversations remains private is fundamental for creating a safe environment. When a person feels assured that their feelings and stories will not be disclosed without their consent, they are more likely to open up and engage authentically. This trust allows for deeper connections and can make the healing process much more effective.

To further uphold confidentiality, professionals might consider anonymizing shared stories or experiences in training or case discussions. This helps to maintain the dignity of individuals while fostering learning and support within a group setting. Ultimately, respect and trust are foundational for effective communication and healing, making it essential to prioritize confidentiality at all levels of care.

To reinforce the establishment of boundaries and confidentiality, it may be helpful to have regular check-ins with grieving individuals about their comfort levels. This practice fosters open lines of communication and allows for adjustments as needed, promoting a nurturing atmosphere for healing.

14.2 Cultural Sensitivity and Respect

When supporting someone in grief, recognizing and honoring their cultural background is essential. Different cultures have unique ways of expressing loss, mourning, and healing, which deeply influence how individuals experience grief. Ignoring these differences may lead to misunderstandings or cause unintended harm.

For example, some cultures may openly express sorrow through loud wailing, while others encourage quiet reflection or maintain a stoic demeanor. Understanding these variations allows grief support providers to connect more meaningfully and offer comfort that respects the grieving person's values and traditions. Grief itself is a universal experience, yet the ways people navigate it vary widely and are often shaped by cultural beliefs about death and the afterlife.

In some cultures, rituals surrounding death are closely tied to spiritual practices and community involvement, while others may focus on private family ceremonies. Respecting these customs means being aware that grief is not a one-size-fits-all experience. This awareness helps prevent assumptions based on one's own cultural lens and encourages a more compassionate, patient response.

Cultural sensitivity fosters trust, which is needed for effective grief support. Respecting diverse cultural practices during grief counseling begins with listening carefully and without judgment. It is important to ask open-ended questions that invite the grieving person to share their customs and preferences, rather than assuming what is appropriate.

For instance, some traditions may call for specific mourning periods, dietary restrictions, or symbolic acts like lighting candles or visiting graves. Even small acts, such as learning how to pronounce names correctly or understanding the significance of certain colors worn during mourning, can show respect and build rapport. Being attentive to these details helps create a supportive environment where grief can be expressed authentically.

Practically speaking, adapting to cultural differences means being flexible in how support is offered. Some people might prefer group settings to share memories and find collective comfort, while others might choose solitude or one-on-one conversations. When working with families from cultures that involve extended kin networks in mourning rituals, it may be helpful to include several family members in discussions, if appropriate.

14.3 Self-Care for Professionals Supporting Grievers

Sensitivity to language barriers and the use of interpreters, when necessary, also plays a critical role in honoring cultural needs. Accepting that each person's grieving journey is shaped by their heritage encourages thoughtful and personalized support. At times, grief workers will face situations where their own beliefs differ greatly from those of the person they are helping.

In these moments, remaining open-minded and setting aside personal biases is crucial. Showing respect does not require agreement with every practice but does involve creating space where the grieving individual feels heard and valued. This approach reduces feelings of isolation and can promote healing by validating the mourner's cultural identity.

Ultimately, respect is shown through genuine curiosity, humility, and the willingness to learn from others' experiences. One practical way to demonstrate cultural sensitivity is by familiarizing oneself with common practices in the communities served before meeting grieving individuals. This background knowledge can prevent inadvertent offenses and offer insights into meaningful ways to support sorrow and remembrance.

Whenever uncertain, simply asking the person about their cultural or religious traditions related to grief often opens pathways to deeper understanding. Never underestimate the power of respectful questions and attentive listening — they create connection and practicing self-care isn't just about feeling better in the moment; it directly impacts a professional's capacity to work sustainably over time. When working with grievers, it's easy to become absorbed in their pain, which can sometimes lead to emotional exhaustion. Setting boundaries around working hours and emotional involvement creates space to recover and prevents the work from becoming overwhelming.

Small routines, like taking breaks during the day, engaging in activities that bring joy, or practicing mindfulness, can help reset emotional energy. It's also helpful to keep a support system, whether colleagues, friends, or a counselor—who can provide a safe space to process feelings. This ongoing effort builds resilience, allowing professionals to show up fully each time without feeling drained or disconnected.

Recognizing early signs of stress or fatigue lets professionals act sooner, rather than risking burnout. Ultimately, maintaining balance is a vital part of staying engaged and effective in supporting those who are grieving. Implementing clear boundaries starts with understanding one's limits and communicating them gently but firmly.

Professionals benefit from defining their work hours tightly rather than leaving open-ended availability that can lead to overextension. For example, setting specific times to respond to emails or calls ensures work doesn't spill into personal time. Creating physical boundaries, like having a dedicated workspace, helps separate work from personal life.

It's also wise to avoid taking work-related stress home by intentionally engaging in activities that mark the end of a workday, like a walk or a hobby. Developing routines that include regular self-check-ins can help identify when emotional fatigue is building up. This might involve journaling, meditation, or simply pausing to assess how one feels and what support might be needed.

Building in time for self-nurturing activities—such as exercise, hobbies, or quiet reflection—supports emotional replenishment. Additionally, leaning on peer support groups or supervision can provide reassurance and guidance, making it easier to handle difficult emotions and prevent feeling isolated. Having these boundaries and practices in place creates a safety net, allowing professionals to sustain their energy and empathy, even during challenging times.

Another practical tip is to set aside time for personal self-care activities that nourish your body and mind. This could mean scheduling regular exercise, ensure sufficient sleep, or pursuing creative outlets like art or music. Recognizing the signs of feeling overwhelmed—such as irritability, fatigue, or detachment— allows for early intervention before stress accumulates.

It's also helpful to stay connected with trusted friends or family members who can offer perspective and emotional support. Making space for reflection, such as keeping a journal or practicing mindfulness, encourages awareness of one's emotional state and can foster inner calm. Professionals should also consider seeking supervision or mentorship, where they can discuss difficult cases and receive encouragement.

Remember, self-care isn't a luxury; it's a necessary part of preserving your ability to share kindness and understanding with those coping with grief. By establishing routines and boundaries that prioritize well-being, you help ensure your ability to continue supporting others with compassion and presence over the long run.

🌸 Summary of Core Takeaways

1. **Boundaries protect both helper and mourner.** They preserve emotional clarity and build trust.

2. **Confidentiality fosters safety and honesty.** Every shared story is sacred.

3. **Cultural sensitivity transforms support into respect.** Every tradition carries wisdom.

4. **Faith diversity deserves curiosity, not correction.** Love listens more than it speaks.

5. **Self-care sustains compassion.** Healthy helpers create safe healing spaces.

6. **Ethics are love in structure.** Integrity is the invisible backbone of effective grief care.

Chapter 15
Integrating Go Hopeful into a Life of Fulfillment

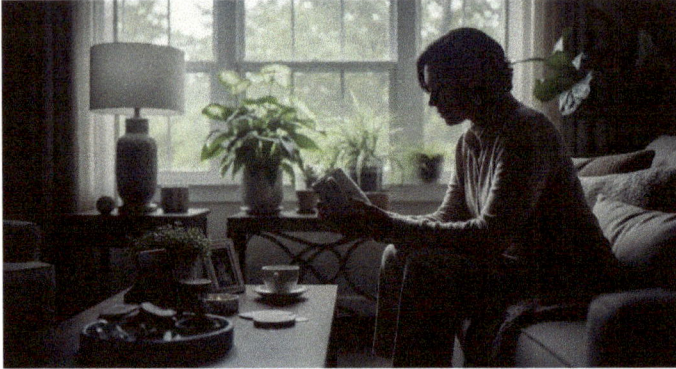

15.1 Transforming Loss into Personal Growth and Wisdom

Confronting loss often sparks a deep journey into one's own thoughts and feelings. When faced with grief, many people begin to question their beliefs, values, and direction in life. This process of introspection can be uncomfortable, yet it is where significant personal growth occurs.

The pain of loss forces individuals to examine what truly matters to them, leading to a clearer understanding of their own strengths and weaknesses. Through this examination, many discover an inner resilience they never knew they had. Grief can strip away the distractions of daily life, leaving just the essence of who we are and what we want.

This can be both frightening and liberating. As people navigate the emotions tied to their loss, they often find themselves developing a greater appreciation for moments of joy and connection. It's not uncommon for individuals to reflect on their relationships with loved ones, fixed beliefs, and previously unexamined aspects of life.

Such reflections may reveal new priorities, changing one's approach to life entirely. Through this painful journey, individuals can build a sense of inner strength. The experience of enduring grief and emerging on the other side nurtures resilience.

People begin to see that they have survived challenges and that their lives can still hold meaning and purpose, even without what they have lost. This realization often leads to a newfound appreciation for life, as well as a determination to live it more fully. Transforming grief into personal growth involves implementing practical strategies that promote healing and clarity.

One effective strategy is to allow yourself to express emotions without judgment. Writing in a journal can be especially helpful in processing complex feelings. By articulating thoughts and emotions on paper, individuals can begin to understand their grief better, which can lead to personal insights.

Engaging in creative outlets such as art, music, or even gardening serves as another beneficial avenue. These activities invite self-expression and can provide solace during tough times. When people direct their grief into something creative, they often uncover deeper insights about themselves and their experiences.

Additionally, it can foster a sense of accomplishment and purpose. Another key strategy is to connect with others who understand the pain of loss. Joining support groups or engaging in counseling can provide a sense of community.

Listening to the stories of others, as well as sharing one's own, can create bonds that are both healing and enlightening. This connection provides reassurance that one is not alone in their grief and can inspire hope when life feels heavy. It is also vital to establish new routines that cultivate a sense of normalcy and purpose.

Simple actions like setting daily goals or participating in community service can spark feelings of accomplishment and joy. Practicing gratitude, even when times are hard, can shift focus from loss to the blessings still present in life. These shifts can help build resilience and embrace a renewed sense of purpose, allowing individuals to honor their loss while continuing to grow and thrive.

Each small step taken during this challenging journey can accumulate into significant transformation. Grief, while painful, holds the potential for profound personal growth. By embracing the journey and exploring strategies that foster resilience, individuals can emerge stronger, wiser, and more in tune with their authentic selves.

15.2 Building a Legacy of Compassion and Understanding

Compassion and understanding are the quiet forces that help us navigate the difficult journey of grief. When someone we care about is gone, the pain can feel overwhelming, and healing often begins with self-compassion—allowing ourselves to feel the full range of emotions without judgment. Understanding, both of our own grief and the grief of others, helps create space for genuine connection.

It reminds us that while each person's experience of loss is unique, shared feelings of sorrow and love can bring people together in powerful ways. This shared understanding honors the memory of those lost by keeping their stories alive in empathetic conversations and acts of remembrance. Grief can make people feel isolated, but it's through compassion that isolation can be softened.

When we respond to ourselves and others with kindness, we lay the groundwork for healing. It is in recognizing the pain of others and validating those feelings without rushing to fix everything that a true legacy of compassion begins. Such a legacy respects the complexity of grief and the time it takes to move through the stages of sorrow, acceptance, and remembrance.

By embracing patience and gentle care, we honor humanity within ourselves and those around us, creating an environment where healing becomes possible. Every act of compassion, no matter how small, has the potential to ripple outward and inspire others. These acts don't need to be grand gestures; sometimes, they are simply listening without interrupting, offering a comforting presence, or remembering a detail about the person who has passed that others may have forgotten.

Understanding is about more than just sympathy; it is about truly seeing the needs of those who grieve and respond with openness and heart. When compassion and understanding are woven into the way we respond to loss, they become the foundation upon which healing and honoring loved ones stand strong. Taking steps to build a lasting legacy of compassion starts with simple actions that show kindness and empathy to those carrying grief.

Sometimes this means reaching out with an honest, easy question like "How are you holding up. " and being prepared to listen without offering solutions. Supporting someone in grief might also look like sharing a meal, helping with everyday tasks, or inviting them into a space where they can express their feelings safely.

These genuine moments of care build trust and remind those grieving that they are not alone in their journey, encouraging them to lean on a community that values their experience. Creating spaces where memories can be shared also helps uphold the legacy of those who have passed on. Memorial gatherings, online tribute pages, or even small acts like planting a tree in someone's honor can serve as tangible reminders of love and loss.

These acts not only celebrate the life of the person who is gone but also allow those left behind to find meaning and purpose in remembering. When communities come together in this way, whether through anniversaries, storytelling, or quiet acts of remembrance, they reinforce bonds and remind everyone that grief is a shared human experience. Kindness extends beyond the immediate circle of family and friends.

Offering support to others outside our immediate network widens the circle of compassion and strengthens the sense of connection. Volunteering with grief support groups or simply checking in on neighbors going through loss encourages empathy to ripple through the community. Through consistent acts of empathy, individuals create a ripple effect that encourages healing in unexpected places.

When kindness becomes part of everyday life, it creates a lasting foundation that honors the memory of those lost by nurturing the well-being of the living. A simple but powerful way to foster these values is to practice self-compassion alongside empathy for others. Recognizing that grief is a process without a clear timeline allows for patience with yourself and those you care about.

Supporting each other with this understanding creates a network of emotional safety that strengthens over time. This network becomes a living legacy where the values of compassion and understanding grow, offering a greater sense of peace amid the difficult emotions that come with loss. Finally, when you feel ready, sharing your own experiences of grief with others can help break down isolation and stigma about loss.

Your story becomes part of a collective memory that validates the feelings of others and encourages compassion on a broader scale. By living compassionately and understanding deeply, you lay bricks in the road toward healing, not just for yourself but for everyone touched by grief.

15.3 Sustaining Healing Practices Over Time

Keeping healing practices alive in everyday routines can make a big difference over time. Simple actions like setting aside a few minutes each morning for breathing exercises, journaling, or a brief meditation can create a sense of stability. These rituals don't have to be lengthy; consistency matters more than duration.

For example, lighting a candle for a few minutes each evening can serve as a moment of reflection, helping to process the day's feelings. Making these practices part of normal activities helps them become habits, which in turn support resilience when facing tough emotions. Small, regular acts can build a foundation of calm that persists even during difficult times, helping you stay grounded and emotionally steady.

Adding variety to routines can prevent rituals from feeling like chores, keeping them engaging and meaningful. Some might find comfort in listening to calming music, while others prefer gentle stretches or a short walk in nature. The goal is to choose activities that suit personal preferences and fit into busy schedules, making it easier to stick with them daily.

Using reminders on a phone or placing notes in visible spots can help reinforce these habits. Over time, these ongoing practices serve as gentle anchors, consistently reminding you of your strength and capacity to heal, even though ongoing challenges. Remember, the key is cultivating habits that feel natural and supportive, not burdensome or forced.

Developing a toolkit of routines that are easy to maintain helps turn healing into a continuous process. Whether it's deep breathing, mindfulness, or expressing gratitude, finding a range of practices allows flexibility. When life gets hectic, having a go-to ritual can provide quick relief from overwhelming feelings.

Tracking your progress or simply acknowledging small successes can boost motivation and make these routines feel more rewarding. Over weeks and months, these small steps add up, slowly strengthening your emotional resilience. The consistency of these practices acts like a steady heartbeat in daily life, supporting ongoing healing and helping to develop a sense of inner stability that persists through ups and downs.

Healing isn't about doing the same thing forever without change. Life shifts, emotions evolve, and what worked yesterday may not fit today. Being willing to adjust your routines keeps them relevant and prevents them from feeling stale or burdensome.

Patience plays a big role because healing is often a gradual process. Sometimes, setbacks happen, and that's normal. Instead of viewing them as failures, recognizing that progress includes ups and downs can help maintain a compassionate outlook.

Encouraging yourself to stay flexible and kind during these times can keep you engaged with your practices and prevent frustration from taking over. Building a support network is also essential. Sharing your journey with friends, family, or a support group can provide encouragement and new perspectives.

Sometimes, talking about your feelings or hearing others' stories can validate your experiences and boost motivation. Encouragement from others creates a sense of community, reminding you that you're not alone in your efforts. Understanding that sustained healing may require different strategies at different stages helps maintain patience.

Having someone to lean on when motivation wanes makes it easier to keep practicing—even when the initial enthusiasm fades—reinforcing the idea that healing is a continuous, shared process. Flexibility and patience go hand in hand, making it easier to stay committed over time. If certain rituals stop feeling helpful, being open to trying new approaches can renew interest and effectiveness.

For example, if meditation no longer appeals, perhaps engaging in creative activities like drawing or gardening could serve as healing outlets. Recognizing that healing is a personal journey means allowing space for change without feeling discouraged. Community support, whether through friends, family, or groups with similar experiences, offers reassurance and accountability.

They can help reinforce the idea that healing is ongoing and that progress comes in small steps. Allowing yourself to adapt and be patient with the process creates a more sustainable path toward emotional stability and resilience that endures beyond immediate needs. One practical tip is to set realistic expectations from the start.

Instead of aiming for perfect consistency, focus on making small, manageable adjustments that feel doable. Celebrate even minor achievements to build confidence. Keep in mind that the ability to adapt and seek support is often what sustains healing practices over time, rather than strict adherence to rigid routines. When storms of emotion come up, turning to your community or your flexible routines can provide the comfort needed to keep moving forward. Trust that the ongoing effort, no matter how small, adds up in meaningful ways and helps create a resilient emotional foundation that can withstand life's inevitable ups and downs.

🌸 Core Takeaways

1. **Grief refines, it doesn't define.** Let clarified values shape small, doable goals.
2. **Compassion is your living legacy.** Self-kindness first; shared kindness next.
3. **Rituals + flexibility = durability.** Keep practices brief, consistent, and adjustable.
4. **Community sustains the long road.** Invite support; offer it, too.
5. **Integration over erasure.** You carry love forward as wisdom, purpose, and grace.

Chapter 16
My Next Chapter After Grieving: A Reflective Guide

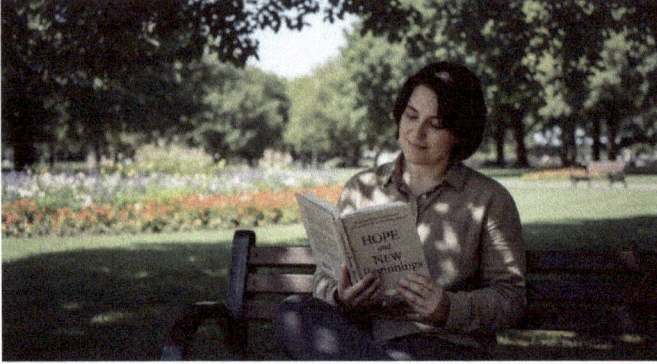

Think of this season like turning a page: the old chapter is written, cherished, and will always be part of your story, but a fresh page is waiting for your words.

16.1 Where I Am Now

- What emotions am I still carrying today?
- What has grief taught me about myself?
- What parts of my old life do I want to carry forward?

A Write a few sentences about how grief has shaped your story so far.

16.2 Honoring What Was Lost

- One memory I treasure deeply is…
- A way I can continue to honor my loved one (or what I lost) is…

- How can I keep their influence alive in my daily life?

Consider creating a small ritual, symbol, or tradition that helps you remember with love instead of only with pain.

16.3 Rediscovering Me

- What brings me peace right now?
- What brings me even small sparks of joy?
- What values feel most important to me as I move forward?

Try making a "Joy List" — even little things like a warm cup of coffee, a walk in nature, or hearing a favorite song.

16.4 Imagining My Next Chapter

- If I could write the next season of my life like a book, what would I want the title to be?
- What new habits, passions, or goals do I feel drawn toward?
- Who do I want by my side in this chapter?

Dream without limits — write freely about the life you want to create.

16.5 Steps Forward

- One small thing I can do this week for my healing is…
- One way I can open myself to new possibilities is…
- One commitment I can make to myself for the future is…

Tiny steps matter. Healing is not a leap, but a series of faithful steps forward.

16.6 Faith, Hope & Purpose

- Where is God (or my faith/values) leading me now?

- How can I turn my pain into purpose?

- What hope do I want to hold onto as I step forward?

Consider writing a prayer, affirmation, or personal declaration for your next chapter.

🌸 Summary of Core Takeaways

1. **Faith shapes how we mourn—but love unites all.**

2. **Rituals create structure, community gives strength, hope brings meaning.**

3. **Learning from different traditions broadens empathy and respect.**

4. **Every faith offers comfort through remembrance and the belief that love endures beyond life.**

Worksheets

The following worksheets cover the various aspects of grief. They are meant to help you work through your grief journey.

1. Handling Anger Worksheet
2. Handling Fear Worksheet
3. Handling Being Hopeful & Resilient Worksheet
4. Handling Regret Worksheet
5. Handling Feeling Overwhelmed Worksheet
6. Handling Your Self-Care Worksheet
7. Handling Loneliness & Sadness Worksheet
8. Handling Your Questions for God Worksheet

Handling Anger Worksheet

1. Recognizing My Triggers

What situations, people, or events usually make me angry? Example: Being ignored, unfair treatment, running late.

My triggers: _____

2. Spotting Warning Signs

What physical or emotional signs tell me I'm getting angry?

Example: Tight chest, clenched fists, raised voice.

My warning signs: _____

3. My Typical Reactions

When I get angry, what do I usually do? Example: Yell, shut down, walk away, hold it in.

My usual reactions: _____

4. Consequences of My Anger

What happens after I react in anger? Example: Hurt relationships, regret, stress.

My consequences: _____

5. Healthier Coping Strategies

What are some positive ways I can respond instead? Take deep breaths

Count to 10 before speaking Go for a walk

Journal my feelings

My healthy strategies: _____

6. Reframing My Thoughts

Write down one unhelpful angry thought you often have:

"No one ever respects me."

Replace it with a calmer, more balanced thought:

"This situation is frustrating, but I can explain my needs calmly."

My reframed thought: _____

7. Taking Responsibility

When I hurt others with anger, how can I make it right? Apologize sincerely

Take responsibility for my words/actions

My repair step: _____

8. Long-Term Anger Management Goals

What new habits do I want to build?

Example: Daily relaxation practice, weekly check-in with emotions.

Tip: Use this worksheet whenever you feel anger building, or as a weekly check-in to track your progress.

Handling Fear Worksheet

1. **Identifying My Fears**

   - What situations, people, or thoughts trigger fear in me?

     o Example: Public speaking, failure, losing someone, rejection.

     o My fears: _____

2. **How Fear Shows Up in My Body**

   - What physical signs tell me I'm afraid?

   o Example: Racing heart, sweaty palms, shallow breathing, tense muscles.

   o My signs: _____

3. **My Typical Reactions to Fear**

   - What do I usually do when I feel afraid?

     o Example: Avoid the situation, stay silent, overthink, run away.

     o My reactions: _____

4. **Consequences of My Fear**

   - What happens because of my fear?

     o Example: Missed opportunities, broken trust, low confidence.

     o My consequences: _____

5. **Understanding the Fear**

   - What does this fear protect me from?

     o Example: Fear of failure protects me from embarrassment.

     o My insight: _____

6. Challenging Fearful Thoughts

- Write down one fearful thought you often have:

  o "If I try, I'll fail and everyone will laugh."

    - Replace it with a calmer, more balanced thought:

    o "I may not be perfect, but I can learn and grow from the experience."

    o My new thought: _____

7. Coping Strategies I Can Use

- Healthy ways I can face my fears:

  o Deep breathing or mindfulness

  o Talking it through with someone I trust

  o Breaking the situation into smaller steps

  o Reminding myself of past victories

  o My coping tools: _

8. Building Courage

- What is one small step I can take toward facing my fear?

  o Example: Practice my speech in front of a mirror.

  o My next step: _____

9. Long-Term Goals

- How do I want to handle fear differently in the future?

  o Example: Respond with courage instead of avoidance.

  o My goals: _

■ Tip: Use this worksheet when fear feels overwhelming, or as a regular practice to build courage and confidence.

Handling Being Hopeful & Resilient Worksheet

1. **Defining Hope in My Life**

- What does *hope* mean to me personally?
  - o Example: Believing things can improve, trusting in God's timing, expecting good in the future.
  - o My definition: _____

2. **Recognizing My Sources of Hope**

- Who or what gives me strength to keep going?
  - o Example: Family, faith, community, memories of past victories.
  - o My sources: _____

3. **Remembering Past Resilience**

- Recall a time I overcame hardship:
  - o What challenge did I face? _____
  - o How did I get through it? _____
  - o What did I learn about myself? _____

4. **Current Challenges**

- What am I struggling with right now?
  - o Example: Grief, uncertainty, health, relationships.
  - o My current challenge: _____

5. **Building Resilient Thoughts**

- Write down one discouraging thought I often have:
  - o "I can't handle this."
- Replace it with a more hopeful one:

- o "This is hard, but I have survived hard things before."
- o My new thought: _____

6. **Strengthening My Coping Tools**

- Healthy strategies I can lean on:
  - o Prayer, journaling, exercise, support groups, creative expression.
  - o My tools: _____

7. **Daily Practices of Hope**

- What small actions help me feel more hopeful?
  - o Example: Gratitude list, morning affirmations, helping others.
  - o My daily hope practice: _____

8. **My Support System**

- Who can I turn to for encouragement and strength?
  - o Example: A trusted friend, family member, pastor, counselor.
  - o My support people: _____

9. **Long-Term Vision**

- If I live with hope and resilience, what will my future look like?
  - o Example: Peaceful, purposeful, stronger, filled with growth.
  - o My vision: _____

Tip: This worksheet works best when revisited regularly — each time you face a setback or need encouragement, it helps remind you of your strength and hope.

Handling Regret Worksheet

1. Naming My Regret

- What do I regret most right now?
    - Example: A decision I made, words I didn't say, time I lost.
    - My regret: _____

2. Feelings Connected to My Regret

- What emotions come up when I think about this regret?
    - Example: Sadness, guilt, shame, disappointment.
    - My emotions: _____

3. The Impact of This Regret

- How has this regret affected my life, relationships, or self-esteem?
    - Example: Holding me back, keeping me stuck in the past.
    - My impact: _____

4. Lessons Learned

- What has this regret taught me about myself or life?
    - Example: I value honesty, I need to take chances sooner.
    - My lessons: _____

5. Reframing the Story

- How can I look at this regret in a new way?
    - Example: Instead of "I failed," think "I learned."
    - My reframed story: _____

6. **Making Amends (if possible)**

- Is there a step I can take to repair the past or bring closure?
    - Example: Apologize, write a letter, express gratitude, let go.
    - My action step: _____

7. **Self-Forgiveness**

- Write one statement of forgiveness toward yourself:
    - "I forgive myself for not knowing then what I know now."
    - My forgiveness statement: _____

8. **Moving Forward**

- What's one healthy way I can use this regret to grow?
    - Example: Make better choices, be more present, take more risks.
    - My growth step: _____

9. **Long-Term Goal**

- How do I want to respond to regrets in the future?
    - Example: With compassion and acceptance instead of self-punishment.
    - My goal: _____

Tip: Regret can be a teacher, not a prison. Use this worksheet to turn past pain into wisdom for your future

Handling Feeling Overwhelmed Worksheet

1. **Naming the Overwhelm**

   - What situation(s) are overwhelming me right now?

     o Example: Too many responsibilities, grief, financial stress.

     o My overwhelm: _____

2. **My Stress Signals**
   - How does overwhelm show up in my body?

     o Example: Headaches, tense shoulders, fatigue.

     o My body signals: _

   - How does overwhelm affect my emotions?

     o Example: Irritability, sadness, anxiety.

     o My emotional signs: _____

3. **Breaking It Down**

   - Write down all the tasks, worries, or situations causing stress:

   _____

   _____

   _____

   - Circle the ones I *can* control. Cross out the ones I *cannot* control.

4. **Prioritizing What Matters**

   - What needs my attention first? _____

   - What can wait? _____

   - What can I delegate or ask help with? _____

5. **Coping in the Moment**

   - Quick calming tools I can use right now:
     ☐ Deep breathing

☐ Grounding exercise (5 things I see, 4 I touch, 3 I hear…)

☐ Short walk/stretch

☐ Journaling

☐ Prayer/meditation

    o My chosen tool:
    _____

6. Shifting My Thoughts

- Overwhelming thought I'm having: _____

- A more balanced thought I can choose instead: _____

7. Support System

- Who can I talk to about how I'm feeling? _____

- One person I can ask for practical help: _____

8. Next Small Step

- What is *one small step* I can take today to ease this feeling?

    o Example: Make a to-do list, send one email, rest.

    o My small step: _____

9. Self-Care Check

- Have I eaten, rested, and hydrated today? ☐ Yes ☐ No

- What's one kind thing I can do for myself tonight? _

Tip: When overwhelm feels big, focus on the *next right step* rather than the whole mountain. Small steps add up to relief.

Handling Your Self-Care Worksheet

1. My Current Self-Care Check-In

- How am I feeling physically right now? ____

- How am I feeling emotionally right now? ___

- How am I feeling spiritually/mentally right now? ___

2. Daily Basics

- Did I get enough sleep last night? ☐ Yes ☐ No

- Did I eat nourishing meals today? ☐ Yes ☐ No

- Did I drink enough water? ☐ Yes ☐ No

- Did I move/stretch my body? ☐ Yes ☐ No

3. Emotional & Mental Care

- Things that bring me peace: _

- Things that bring me joy: ____

- How I usually respond to stress: ____

4. Social & Relational Care

- People who support me: ____

- Someone I want to connect with this week: _

- One boundary I need to set: _

5. Spiritual / Inner Care

- Practices that ground me (prayer, meditation, reflection): ___

- Gratitude list (3 things I'm thankful for today):

    1. _____
    2. _____
    3. _____

6. **Fun & Play**

- Activities that make me smile: _____

7. **Self-Compassion**

- A kind thing I can say to myself today: _____

- One way I can forgive myself or let go of pressure: _

8. **My Self-Care Plan**

- This week, I will prioritize: __

- One daily habit I want to improve: __

- My commitment to myself: __

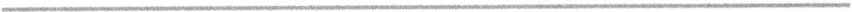

Tip: Review this worksheet weekly — it will show patterns and remind you where you need to refill your "self-care tank."

Handling Negative Thinking Worksheet

1. **Notice the Thought**

   - What is the negative thought you are having?

   Example: "I always mess things up."

   - Write it down:

   _____

   _____

2. **Check the Evidence**

   - What facts support this thought?

   _____

   - What facts do NOT support this thought?

   _____

   _____

3. **Identify Thinking Traps**

   (Check any that apply)

   ☐ All-or-Nothing Thinking (black C white, no middle ground)

   ☐ Overgeneralizing (assuming "always" or "never")

   ☐ Mind Reading (assuming what others think)

   ☐ Catastrophizing (expecting the worst)

   ☐ Should Statements ("I should... I must...")

   ☐ Personalizing (blaming yourself unfairly)

   ☐ Other: _____

4. Challenge the Thought

- Is this thought 100% true?

- Is there another way to look at it?

- If my friend had this thought, what would I tell them? New balanced thought:

_____

_____

5. Replace with Truth / Positives

- Write a more encouraging or realistic statement:

_____

- List 2–3 strengths, blessings, or truths that counter the negative thought:

    1. _____

    2. _____

    3. _____

6. Action Step

- What small action can I take to move forward in a healthier way?

_____

_____

🌟 *Tip: Keep practicing. The more often you replace negative thoughts with balanced ones, the more natural it becomes.*

📝 Handling Your Questions for God Worksheet

1. What's On My Heart?

- The main question I want to ask God right now is:

_____

- Other questions I've been holding inside:

_____

_____

2. Emotions Behind My Questions

- When I think about these questions, I feel:

☐ Angry ☐ Sad ☐ Confused ☐ Hopeless ☐ Curious ☐ Grateful
- My emotions in my own words: _____

3. What Scripture Says

- A verse that comes to mind about my question:

_____

- How this verse speaks to me (comforts, challenges, or confuses):

_____

_____

4. Listening for God's Voice

- In prayer or quiet reflection, what do I sense God might be saying?

_____

- Does anything in creation, music, or conversation point me toward an answer?

---

5. **Trusting the Unknown**
   - Even if I don't have answers yet, what truth can I hold onto?
     - Example: "God is with me," "God's timing is perfect."
     - My truth: __

6. **My Next Step of Faith**
   - One way I can bring this question to God again (prayer, journaling, worship, talking with a mentor):

   - One act of trust I can take today (even without full answers):

   ---

7. **Gratitude in the Waiting**
   - Three things I can thank God for, even as I wait for answers: 1.
     1. _____
     2. _____
     3. _____

✅ Tip: This worksheet is not about finding immediate answers, but about deepening conversation with God. Sometimes His answers come in whispers, people, or moments over time.

Closing Thoughts

On the planet Earth there is some where between 6 and a half to 8 billion people. None has the same finger print which makes each one of us unique. So is our grief journey unique as no one has exactly the same.

Your story is still being written. Although Grief may be part of your journey, it does not define the whole of it. This next chapter is yours to shape—with love, courage, and hope.

May God help you find that path forward, always keeping your love ones in your heart, as you discover a renewed purpose.

God bless and keep you!

Suggested Reading List

A Grief Observed – C.S. Lewis

Honest reflections of faith shaken and renewed after loss.

Healing After Loss – Martha Whitmore Hickman

Daily meditations for calm reflection through the grieving journey.

It's OK That You're Not OK – Megan Devine

A modern guide that normalizes grief and encourages emotional honesty.

Grieving with Hope – Samuel J. Hodges IV & Kathy Leonard

Combines Scripture with counseling principles to balance faith and feelings.

Good Grief – Granger E. Westberg

A timeless Christian classic outlining ten stages of healthy mourning.

When God Doesn't Make Sense – Dr. James Dobson

Offers spiritual grounding when tragedy challenges belief.

Experiencing Grief – H. Norman Wright

Short, faith-based reflections perfect for those feeling spiritually numb.

Understanding Your Grief – Dr. Alan Wolfelt

Ten touchstones for emotional healing, blending heart and psychology.

The Grief Recovery Handbook – John W. James & Russell Friedman

A practical step-by-step guide to complete "unfinished business" with loss.

A Grace Disguised – Jerry Sittser

Profound reflections on how loss can enlarge the soul rather than destroy it.

Dark Clouds, Deep Mercy – Mark Vroegop

Teaches the biblical art of lament — expressing pain honestly before God.

The Grieving Brain – Mary-Frances O'Connor

Reveals how grief physically rewires the brain and why healing takes time.

Life After Loss – Bob Deits

A steady, structured guide that blends faith, counseling, and real-life stories.

How to Live When a Loved One Dies – Thich Nhat Hanh

Gentle, mindful reflections on presence, love, and letting go.

The Journey Through Grief – Alan D. Wolfelt

Explores the four phases of grief with deep compassion and practical wisdom.

Shattered: Surviving the Loss of a Child – Gary Roe

Deeply empathetic guide for those facing devastating loss and identity rebuilding.

From Grief to Healing – Tom Zuba

A holistic approach to living fully again after loss, centered on meaning and love.

Tear Soup – Pat Schwiebert & Chuck DeKlyen

A beautifully illustrated parable on giving yourself permission to grieve your way.

Renegade Grief – Carla Fernandez

Encourages creative, nontraditional healing rituals and redefining remembrance.

The One Year Book of Hope – Nancy Guthrie

A devotional journey of faith renewal, offering daily comfort and perspective.